A Glimpse into Medical Practice among Jews around 1500

A Glimpse into Medical Practice among Jews around 1500

Latin-German Pharmaceutical Glossaries in Hebrew Characters Extant in Ms Leiden, Universiteitsbibliotheek, Cod. Or. 4732/1 (SCAL 15), fols. 1a–17b

Edited by

Gerrit Bos
Klaus-Dietrich Fischer

BRILL

LEIDEN | BOSTON

Cover illustration: Collective volume with texts in Hebrew and German: *Shemot ha-Asavim*; and other texts; Ms Leiden, Universiteitsbibliotheek, Cod. Or. 4732/1 (SCAL 15), fol. 2a, reproduced under Creative Commons CC BY License.

The Library of Congress Cataloging-in-Publication Data is available online at http://catalog.loc.gov
LC record available at http://lccn.loc.gov/2021001658

Typeface for the Latin, Greek, and Cyrillic scripts: "Brill". See and download: brill.com/brill-typeface.

ISBN 978-90-04-45913-7 (hardback)
ISBN 978-90-04-45938-0 (e-book)

This book is printed on acid-free paper and produced in a sustainable manner.

Contents

Transliteration System

Hebrew letter	Name	Transliteration sign
א	Alef	ʾ
ב	Bet	B
ב׳	Vet	V
ג	Gimel	G
ג׳	Ğimel	Ğ
ד	Dalet	D
ה	He	H
ו	Waw	W
ז	Zayin	Z
ח	Ḥet	Ḥ
ט	Ṭet	Ṭ
י	Yod	Y
כ/ך	Kaf	K
ל	Lamed	L
מ/ם	Mem	M
נ/ן	Nun	N
ס	Samekh	S
ע	Ayin	ʿ
פ/ף	Pe	P
פ׳	Fe	F
צ/ץ	Ṣade	Ṣ
ק	Qof	Q
ר	Resh	R
ש	Shin	Š
ת	Tav	T

Hebrew vowel sign	Name	Transliteration sign
ָ	qamaṣ	a
ַ	pataḥ	a
ֵ	ṣere	e
ִ	ḥiriq	i
וֹ	Waw & ḥolam	Wo
וּ	Waw & shuruq	Wu
ֻ	qubuṣ	u
ְ	shwa	ə

Introduction

Few non-specialists will realize that, until a short while ago, all medicines were natural because chemistry had not progressed sufficiently to allow for the creation of chemical compounds useful for treating diseases.* Among the three kingdoms of nature—as they were called; namely, plants, animals, and minerals—plants were by far the most important, as a glance at the two most important works from antiquity by Dioscorides (first century AD) and Galen (second century AD) will show. Galen's work *On Simple Drugs* devotes three books to plants (bks. 6–8), one to minerals (bk. 9) and the last two to products deriving from animals (bks. 10 and 11). Even in our lifetime, botany (for medical purposes) was part of the regular medical curriculum in Germany and doubtless in many other countries as well. It is clear that nature itself would be the best place to be introduced to medicinal plants, led by an expert, something that is impossible when a particular plant does not grow where you happen to live, which applies not just to exotic imports.[1] The invention of the printing press provided the opportunity for depicting plants much more faithfully than illustrations in manuscripts had allowed for and at a much more affordable price. Pictures are, of course, a much better guide than verbal descriptions like the ones Dioscorides provided, or just plant names, because one name might refer to different plants, or a given plant would have more than one name, in Latin or in the vernacular. Still, a recipe in a medical book that was not an illustrated herbal would only use that particular name, at best alongside a synonym. It must be kept in mind that medicines would normally be prepared by the healer or physician and not an apothecary or pharmacist, because their number increased very slowly and they would only be found in places where there was sufficient business.

Jewish physicians, like Jews in general, lived in a world of their own and, while not rarely respected and sought after by gentiles, had neither regular access to medical education in Christian universities because of their religion, nor to medical writings in Latin, given that the study of Latin was not part of their education. This explains not only the translation of Latin medical works into Hebrew made in the High and Late Middle Ages for the use by Jewish

* We thank Stephen Lawrence, Cambridge, for drawing our attention to the manuscript with these lists; Dr. Arnoud Vrolijk, Curator of Oriental Manuscripts and Rare Books at Leiden Universiteitsbibliotheek, for providing us with high-resolution digital prints of the manuscript; and Felix Hedderich for checking the proofs.

1 O. Brunfels, *Herbarum vivae eicones ad naturae imitationem, summa cum diligentia & artificio*

 | DOI:10.1163/9789004459380_002

physicians in different countries, but also their translation into various vernacular languages (but still written in Hebrew characters) and thus only intended for a specific area.

The need for glossaries, brought about by the vast amount of synonyms, especially where plants were concerned, had been felt for a long time; it can be documented at least from the time of Dioscorides. In the High and Late Middle Ages, the most famous medical glossaries were the *Alphita*,[2] followed by Simon of Genoa's much more comprehensive *Clavis sanationis* at the turn of the thirteenth century,[3] and, even later, the work of Matthaeus Silvaticus[4] (1285–1342) that is based on Simon. As far as pharmacognostic literature is concerned, the (anonymous) *Circa instans*[5] had probably achieved the widest circulation. All of these works were naturally composed in Latin and, with the exception of the *Alphita*, lack modern critical editions and have to be used as incunabula or in manuscript.[6]

Our attempts to link the two glossaries presented here with these well-known works were unsuccessful, which is to be regretted especially because such a link could have helped with clarifying entries in the glossaries that are mangled and therefore cannot be understood and corrected. In many cases, this may have been because the rendering of Latin and German words in Hebrew characters made it impossible to establish their meaning with any degree of certainty and this applies even more to German than to Latin words. Although the monumental *Wörterbuch der deutschen Pflanzennamen* (*Dictionary of German Plant Names*) compiled by the German botanist Heinrich Marzell (1885–1970) is a reference work of the greatest value, we discovered to our surprise many German plant names that are not listed there, which on the other hand testifies to the value of the two glossaries edited here for further research.

Since antiquity and the Middle Ages, the fact that one single name may refer to many different plants has not changed. This implies that even a correctly reconstructed Latin name will not necessarily help us with the German equivalent presented in our glossaries. The specification of the degree of a certain drug—if given—may, however, at times provide a clue. Galen had tried

---

effigiatae, una cum Effectibus earundem, in gratiam veteris illius & iamiam renascentis Herbariae Medicinae, per Othonem Brunfelsium recens editae, Argentorati 1532.

2 Compiled perhaps in the first half of the thirteenth century (García González, 49); full references to be found in ch. 'Reconstruction of Latin and German Terms' below.

3 See www.simonofgenoa.org for the text.

4 *Opus pandectarum medicine*, [Bononiae] 1474, GW M42128.

5 Cf. Ventura below.

6 Perhaps the most convenient site for access is Bayerische Staatsbibliothek München, Digitale Sammlungen.

to establish a solid theoretical basis for applying drugs in therapy by further dividing the four qualities hot, cold, wet, and dry into four distinct degrees to be determined by the senses (especially by taste and touch).[7] Galen's approach had a real impact only in Islamic medicine. When with the translation of works written in Arabic into Latin this system of degrees began to be received in the Latin west (the earliest and perhaps most important work in this respect being Constantine the African's *Liber graduum*, written at the end of the eleventh century), it became prevalent in the western Middle Ages. Our glossaries do, in many cases, specify the property of the drug indicating a degree, which may help with its identification. Nevertheless, since opinions regarding qualities and degrees not seldom vary, they will not necessarily help in all cases of ambiguity.

1 Ms Leiden, Universiteitsbibliotheek, Cod. Or. 4732/1 (SCAL 15)

The following edition consists of two unique separate glossaries of medico-botanical terms in Latin and German in Hebrew characters, which are extant in the unique Ms Leiden, Universiteitsbibliotheek, Cod. Or. 4732/1 (SCAL 15). The first glossary covers fols. 1a–11b and the second one fols. 11b–17b.[8] The Ms was copied in the fifteenth/sixteenth century in an Ashkenazi script. Jewish physicians probably used these kinds of lists, written in Hebrew, for the acquisition of herbs at the local market or elsewhere for the composition of the medications they needed. In general, the writing of the Ms is clear and can be read without problems; however, several entries on fols. 11a and 14b can only be read partially due to the fact that the ink from the counter side (fols. 10b and 13a) has come through the thin parchment and left blotches on the text written there. In spite of the general clarity of the script, several entries are hard to identify as they suffer from scribal errors.

7 G. Harig, *Bestimmung der Intensität im medizinischen System Galens: Ein Beitrag zur theoretischen Pharmakologie, Nosologie und Therapie* in der Galenischen Medizin, Berlin 1974 (Schriften zur Geschichte und Kultur der Antike, vol. 11).

8 Cf. M. Steinschneider, *Catalogus Codicum Hebraeorum Bibliothecae Academiae Lugduno-Batavae*, Leiden 1858, p. 372; A. van der Heide, *Hebrew Manuscripts of Leiden University Library*, Leiden 1977, p. 64. See also J.P. Rothschild, "Remarques sur la tradition manuscrite du glossaire Hébreux-Italien du commentaire de Moïse de Salerne au *Guide des Egarés* (en Appendices, note sur les glossaires médicaux hébreux; Liste de manuscrits hébreux contenant des glossaires)," in: *Lexiques bilingues dans les domaines philosophiques et scientifiques*, ed. by J. Hamesse and D. Jacquart, Turnhout 2001, pp. 67–68.

The first glossary is entitled שמות העשבים (Plant Names) and consists of 381 entries that are alphabetically arranged. It runs from fol. 1a until 11b and ends with the letter *Resh*. However, it is not incomplete as several terms starting with the penultimate letter *Shin* (that follows *Resh*) feature under the letter *Samekh*, and the letter *Tav*, the last letter of the Hebrew alphabet, has not been used to transliterate Latin or German -t-. For the transliteration of this letter, the author used Hebrew *Ṭet*. In addition to the plant names in Latin and the parallel terms in German, the first list generally provides us with information (in Hebrew) about the degrees of heat and cold of individual ingredients and in a few cases it provides some additional information for which the *Alphita* seems to have been an important source.

The second glossary, consisting of 193 entries, simply starts with אלפא בית אחר (Another alphabet[ical list]) and runs from fol. 11b until 17b.[9] Except for an occasional entry, this list does not inform us about the powers of the drugs, nor about their healing properties. However, the explanations in Hebrew are generally longer.

Most of the German terms in Hebrew characters are unvowelized and the vocalisations admit a variety depending on region and time and/or source(s) they were derived from.

These two glossaries are rare examples of botanical terms in Latin and German in Hebrew characters that have been preserved. The only other examples we know about are two glossaries preserved in Ms Oxford, Bodleian Library, Opp. 180 (cat. Neubauer 2134) on fols. 149a–156b and 156b–159a, with parallel terms and/or explanations in German.[10] The foreword to the latter glossary on fol. 156b is especially interesting as the compiler stresses the need for such glossaries since most glossaries provide the names of the drugs in Arabic, but not in German: 'These are synonyms (botanical terms) that I tried as well as I could to render from Arabic into German. I put them in alphabetical order for the benefit of the reader. Physicians need such [lists with German synonyms] urgently since most of the older [glossaries] only contain drug names in Arabic and Latin. Generally, physicians are not familiar with these.'

---

9 Fol. 16b does not belong to the list, as it has a variety of recipes written in a different hand.

10 Cf. A. Neubauer, *Catalogue of the Hebrew Manuscripts in the Bodleian Library*, Oxford 1886, repr. 1994. And: *Supplement of Addenda and Corrigenda* compiled under the direction of M. Beit-Arié and edited by R.A. May, Oxford 1994.

2 Some Peculiar Features of the Latin-German Terminology in Hebrew Characters

Some peculiar features of the way in which Latin words appear in Hebrew letters in these glossaries must be mentioned at the outset. Vocalization is rare, but where it occurs, it not rarely runs contrary to what we expect. While in Medieval Latin spelling variants in the body of words naming medicinal plants etc. are common (cf. DMLBS and MLW), seeing regular Latin words ending in *-on* or *-om* (ון- or ום-) is unusual, even more so when they are easily identifiable as a morpheme (like *-arum* for the genitive plural of the first declension) that any person with a basic knowledge of Latin, like the authors of our two lists, would have been familiar with. Such an ending *-on* will also not represent the ending of originally Greek words that had -ον in Greek, as our examples show. We preferred preserving this irregularity with a view to other similar texts that come to light in the future. Even more puzzling is the letter א (*Aleph*) at the end of German words where it does not belong and does not stand for any vowel, be it in late Middle High German or an earlier form of the language—a silent א! The sound /f/ in Latin and German words would regularly be written פ, a Hebrew letter that is likewise used for /p/. In other cases, ב׳, transliterated as V, again renders the /f/ sound, which in contemporary German texts occurs as v, e.g., in 'von'. In accordance with contemporary usage, we do not distinguish in Latin words between *u* as a vowel or as a consonant, and write *u* in all cases. Similarly, the spelling *-ci-* is preferred over classical *-ti-*, as was the case in the later Middle Ages, when our glossaries were compiled. In Hebrew, Latin *c* in *ce* or *ci* or *cy* is usually spelled צ; the rarer alternative spelling with ס may possibly reflect an origin in a Romance-speaking area. Again in keeping with contemporary usage, classical Latin *-ae-*, often found as an ending for the genitive or the plural of first declension nouns, is written *e*, while the Hebrew often has י (*Yod*) (word final *-ce* occurs as both צי and סי). The choice whether י is rendered as *i* or *e* is made according to other attestations of the word and should be carefully examined by Germanists.

In many cases, the Latin-German terms in Hebrew characters deviate from what is an acceptable variation to such a degree that emendations had to be introduced, rather than preserving utterly strange forms that cannot have been at all current and understood by medical practitioners, or apothecaries, or sellers of *materia medica*. These emendations concern both the Latin and German terms. The deviations from the regular forms that we would expect can only be explained as the result of a process of transmission during which mistakes were being made and the knowledge necessary for correcting such mistakes was lacking. The numerous writing errors in the case of the Latin lemmata and their German translations suggest that these are indeed writing errors and not alternative forms, although we cannot be absolutely certain. The only method of verification is that of the transmission of these unusual terms in which we look at two aspects, whether the unusual form is transmitted in other sources, or features frequently or at least more than once in a work that was distributed widely, such as the *Circa instans* or *Alphita*.[11]

Sometimes, the text transmitted in our only witness has defied all attempts at divining what may be hidden, especially when neither the Latin nor, in cases of difficulty with the Latin, the German equivalent given would provide a clue. In such cases, we write '*uncertain*' and invite our readers to come up with a solution.

The two glossaries will be presented in the following manner:

(a) an edition of the Hebrew text of both glossaries with a transliteration of the Latin and German terms (see transliteration system).

(b) a reconstruction of the Latin and the German terms (entries in Glossary 2 are marked with ″)

- column 1: Latin entries both regularized and as they appear in the glossary (between brackets); word forms marked with an asterisk (*) were not encountered in the dictionaries we consulted, or not with the required meaning;
- column 2: German entries as they feature in the glossary;
- column 3: regularized forms of the German entries as they can be found in the German dictionary of Jacob and Wilhelm Grimm. Following their usage, German nouns are not capitalised and sz is used for ß and ss. Many plant names, e.g., 'weiszdistel,' consist of a combination of adjective + noun; in Grimm's dictionary, these are usually listed under the noun;
- column 4: editors' notes.

(c) Hebrew, Latin, and German indexes.

11 Many variant readings for the German terminology feature in W.F. Daems, *Nomina simplicium medicinarum ex synonymariis medii aevi collecta: Semantische Untersuchungen zum Fachwortschatz hoch- und spätmittelalterlicher Drogenkunde*, Leiden-New York-Köln 1993, and for the Latin and Romance terms in G. Mensching, *La sinonima delos nonbres delas medeçinas griegos e latynos e arauigos*, estudio y edición crítica, Madrid 1994.

Edition of Glossary 1 (fols. 1a–11b)

שמות העשבים 1a
(Plant Names)

[1] אפטריום ב״א ווילדא זילבא חם בראשו׳ ויבש בשני
'PṬRYWM; German WWYLD' ZYLB'; hot in the first degree and dry in the second

[2] אימבליצי ב״א ווינשטיין
'YMBLYṢY; German WWYNŠṬYYN

[3] אנדיביי ב״א וויזא דישטלא קר ויבש במעלה השני
'NDYBYY; German WWYZ' DYŠṬL'; cold and dry in the second degree

[4] אמילא ב״א אלנט חם בשני ולח בראשון
'MYL' [read: 'NWL']; German 'LNṬ; hot in the second degree and moist in the first

[5] איפיטימי וטימי׳ ב׳ מינים הם חם ויבשים במעלה הראשון
'YPYṬYMY and ṬYMY'; two species; they are hot and dry in the first degree

[6] איפורשיון הוא גומא חזק ח״ו במעלה ג׳
'YPWRŠYWN [read: YPWRBYWN]; i.e., strong gum; hot and [dry] in the third degree

[7] איפטיסי ב״א לעבר קרוט ח״ו במעלה א׳
'YPṬYSY; German L'BR QRWṬ; hot and [dry] in the first degree

[8] אזוסטום ב״א גליצישטיין הירוק ח״ו ב״ד
'ZWSṬWM; German green GLYṢYŠṬYYN; hot and [dry] in the fourth degree

[9] אליברום ב״א ניזא ווירצא שחורה
'LYBRWM; German NYZ' WWYRṢ'; black

[10] אזולא ה׳ מיני⟨ם⟩ מינורא ארמיור ארמנדיאור מזדדיון
'ZWL'; five species MYNWR'; 'RMYWR [read: MYWR]; 'RMNDY'WR; MZDDYWN

 | DOI:10.1163/9789004459380_003

[11] א⟨.⟩ולא ח״ו במעלה ג׳
’[.]WL’ [read: ’NWL’]; hot and [dry(?)] in the third degree

[12] אירוקא הוא ארוקל והוא חרדל ⟨...⟩ ח״ו ב״ג
’YRWQ’; it is ’RWQL and this is mustard [...]; hot and [dry] in the third degree

[13] איבולש ב״א אטיך קר ויבש
’YBWLŠ; German ’ṬYK; cold and dry

[14] אנצייני ב״א אֶנְצְיון ח״ו ב״ג
’NṢYYNY [read: ’NṢY’NI]; German ’eNəṢəYWN; hot and [dry] in the third degree

[15] ארמודקטלוש ב״א האלא הובט ח״ו ב״ג
’RMWDQṬLWŠ; German H’L’ HWBṬ; hot and [dry] in the third degree

[16] אישפא ב״א איזופא ח״ו בשלישי
’YŠP’; German ’YZWP’; hot and [dry] in the third degree

1b [17] אריאוש ב״א בלא ליליין ח״ו ב״ב
’RY’WŠ; German BL’ LYLYYN; hot and [...] in the second degree

[18] אניפרום ב״א דור בירן ח״ו ב״ב
’NYPRWM [read: ’YNYPRWM]; German DWR [read: WKLDR] BYRN; hot and [...] in the second degree

[19] אזימום ב״א בזיליין זאמא חם ויבש
’ZYMWM [read: ’WZYMWM]; German BZYLYYN Z’M’; hot and dry

[20] אזפיום קר ויבש ברביעי והוא גומא
’ZPYWM [read: ’WPYWM]; cold and dry in the fourth degree; i.e., GWM’

[21] אוריגנום ב״א דושטא ח״ו ב״ג
’WRYGNWM; German DWŠṬ’; hot and [dry] in the third degree

[22] אוקשיפנציא ב״א זורא אנפרא ק״ו ב״ב
’WQŠYPNṢY’ [read: ’WQŠYLPṢY’]; German ZWR’ ’NPR’; cold and [...] in the second degree

[23] אורטיאום ב״א גערשטין מעלא ק״ו ב״ב
ʾWRṬYʾWM; German GʿRŠṬYN MʿLʾ; cold and [...] in the second degree

[24] אושיש דאקורדי אצערבי ב״א ביצכן הנמצ׳ בלב האייל
ʾWŠYŠ DʾQWRDY ʾṢʿRBY; German BYṢKN [read: BYNKN] that can be found in the heart of the deer

[25] אושיט שיפיי קר ויבש
ʾWŠYṬ [read: ʾWŠYŠ] ŠYPYY; cold and dry

[26] אוליבנום ב״א ווירוך חם ב״ב
ʾWLYBNWM; German WWYRWK; hot in the second degree

[27] אפי ב״א אֶפא חם ב״ב
ʾPY [read: ʾPYY]; German ʾePʾ; hot in the second degree

[28] אזרי ב״א הזל ווירצא חם במעל׳ ג׳
ʾZRY; German HZL WWYRṢʾ; hot in the third degree

[29] אפורב״י הוא גומ׳ ח״ו בד׳
ʾPWRVY; i.e., gum; hot and [dry] in the fourth degree

[30] אניטי ב״א טִימְא חם ב״ב
ʾNYṬY; German ṬiYMəʾ [read: ṬiYLəʾ]; hot in the second degree

[31] אניזי ב״א אניש חם ב״ב
ʾNYZY; German ʾNYŠ; hot in the second degree

[32] אליפטי מושקדי הוא מרקח
ʾLYPṬY MWŠQDY; i.e., a compound

[33] אפופנק הוא גומא׳ חם ב״מ(?) ג׳
ʾPWPNQ [read: ʾPWPNQŠ]; i.e., gum; hot in the third degree

[34] אפשנטין וי״א אפשנצין ב״א וורארא
ʾPŠNṬYN [read: ʾPŠNṬYWN]; and some say: ʾPŠNṢYN [read: ʾPŠNṢYWN]; German WWRʾRʾ [read: WWRMWṬʾ]

2a[1] [35] אורוצייקום הוא גומ׳ חם ב״ב
'WRWṢYYQWM; i.e., gum; hot in the second degree

[36] אנא קרדי ב״א חלפנט לושא חם ב״ג
'N' QRDY; German ḤLPNṬ LWŠ'; hot in the third degree

[37] אייצי ב״א ברבטורא חם ב״ג
'YYṢY; German BRBṬWR'; hot in the third degree

[38] אזורי ב״א געלא ליליין חם ב״ב
'ZWRY [read: 'QWRY]; German G'L' LYLYYN; hot in the second degree

[39] ארישטלונגי ב״א אושטור לוציון חם ב״ב
'RYŠṬLWNGY [read: 'RYŠṬLWNGY']; German 'WŠṬWR [read: 'WŠṬYR] LWṢYWN; hot in the second degree

[40] אמיאי הוא זרע שחור חם ב״ב
'MY'Y; this is a black seed; hot in the second degree

[41] אמומי ב״א ווילדא פיטור חם ב״ב
'MWMY; German WWYLD' PYṬWR [read: PYṬR(?)]; hot in the second degree

[42] אוריצטימוש ב״א כסף חי קר ב״ב
'WRYṢṬYMWŠ; German [read: Hebrew] KSP ḤY; cold in the second degree

[43] אלברום מרגריטום ב״א דגולברוט
'LBRWM MRGRYṬWM [read: MRGRYṬRWM]; German DGWLBRWṬ [read: DNGLKRWṬ(?)]

[44] אירבי פּוֹרְפּוֹרָטִי ב״א יהנס קרוט חם ב״ג
'YRBY PWoRəPWoRaṬiY; German YHNS QRWṬ; hot in the third degree

[45] אשקווֹנטי ב״א קעמלין קרוט הווא חם ב״א
'ŠQWWoNṬY [read: 'ŠQWWiNNṬY]; German Q'MLYN QRWṬ HWW'; hot in the first degree

---

1 In the middle of the top of fol. 2a we find, as a sort of header, a single term written in the same script: אפושטוליקון. In the left margin we find two additional entries written in a different

[46] אליברום ב״א ניזא וורץ חם ב״ד
'LYBRWM; German NYZ' WWRṢ; hot in the fourth degree

[47] אַפְּשֵׁנְצְיוֹ ב״א וורמוטא חם ב״ד ויש קור׳ אַסִינְצוּ
'aPəŠeNəṢəYWo [read: 'aPəŠeNəṢəYWuN]; German WWRMWṬ'; hot in the fourth degree; some read: 'aSiNəṢWu [read: 'aSiNəṢWuN]

[48] איפיריקון ב״א יהנש קרוט חם ב״ב
'YPYRYQWN; German YHNŠ QRWṬ; hot in the second degree

[49] אברוטנום ב״א שטבא וורץ חם ב״ב
'BRWṬNWM; German ŠṬB' WWRṢ; hot in the second degree

[50] ארמודיקטום ב״א היילא הובטא חם ב״ב
'RMWDYQṬWM [read: 'RMWDQṬYLWM]; German HYYL' HWBṬ'; hot in the second degree

[51] איריש ב״א ליליין וויץ
'YRYŠ; German LYLYYN WWYṢ

[52][2] אפטיקוֹם ב״א לעבר קרוט
'PṬYQWoM; German L'BR QRWṬ

[53] ארטמיזייא ב״א ביבוש חם ב״ב 2b
'RṬMYZYY' [read: 'RṬMYZY']; German BYBWŠ; hot in the second degree

[54] אוזימום ב״א פריזיליין חם ב״א
'WZYMWM; German PRYZYLYYN; hot in the first degree

[55] ארמונייקום הוא מלח סדומי חם מאד
'RMWNYYQWM; i.e., salt[3] of Sodom that is very hot

---

script: אֲלֵיגַטוּלִיאַה דרך(?) מוך להריון (alegatulia (electuary?) as a pessary [to prevent] conception) and אַטַנַאקִיאַה (*אַטַנַאסִיאַה) משק׳ להריון (athanasia: a potion for pregnancy(?)).

2 The entry features at the bottom of the folio in a bold, larger script; it was possibly added later on.

3 For "salt of Sodom," see S. Krauss, *Talmudische Archäologie*, Leipzig 1910–1912, vol. 1, p. 119, and p. 501, n. 660; J. Preuss, *Biblical and Talmudic Medicine*, trans. and ed. by F. Rosner, New York 1978, p. 525. It was allegedly so caustic that it could blind the eyes when one would touch them with one's fingers on which it would adhere after the meal. The danger of Sodomite salt is one of the explanations given for the obligation to wash one's hands after meals (מים אחרונים).

[56] אנטימושא ב״א בלי עשא קר ב״ד
'NṬYMWŠ'; German BLY 'Š'; cold in the fourth degree

[57] אכסיא ב״א ריש שאלץ
'KSY'; German RYŠ Š'LṢ

[58] איפוקווישטידוש ב״א פונדוש רוזש חם ב״ב
'YPWQWWYŠṬYDWŠ; German PWNDWŠ RWZŠ [read: HWNDYŠ RWZ']; hot in the second degree

[59] אירביי בלאצי ב״א מילטא מוטר חם ב״ב
'YRBYY BL'ṢY; German MYLṬ' MWṬR; hot in the second degree

[60] אמידום הוא לחם קר ב״א
'MYDWM; i.e., "bread;" cold in the first degree

[61] אורובי ב״א וויקין חם ב״א
'WRWBY; German WWYQYN; hot in the first degree

[62] איריאוש ב״א וויש ליליין חם ב״ג
'YRY'WŠ; German WWYŠ LYLYYN; hot in the third degree

[63] אישפרגי הוא זרע קר ב״א ⟨...⟩ והיא נקי׳ והזכר נקר׳ ברושקי
'YŠPRGY; it is a cold seed; German [...]; it is female; the male variety is called BRWŠQY

[64] אורטיסי ב״א נסלא חם ב״ג
'WRṬYSY; German NSL'; hot in the second degree

[65] אשפודיום ב״א גברנט חלפין צנא קר ב״ד(?)
'ŠPWDYWM; German GBRNṬ ḤLPYN ṢN'; cold in the fourth(?) degree

[66] אַשְׁקְוֶולוי ב״א מֵר צוובל חם ב״ג
'aŠəQWWeLWY; German MeR ṢWWBL; hot in the third degree

[67] איב׳יש חם ב״ב
'YVYŠ; hot in the second degree

[68] איבולי ב״א אַרְבְא חם ב״ג
'YBWLY; German 'aRəBə'; hot in the third degree

[69] אזפטדי הוא גומ׳ וקור׳ לו זבל שטן
’ZPṬDY; i.e., gum, it is also called “devil’s dung”

[70] אגריק ב״א הולצא שוומא לו חם ב״ב 3a
’GRYQ; German HWLṢ’ ŠWWM’; hot in the second degree

[71] אלוואי איפטיסי הוא גומ׳ והוא שחור ומשלשל
’LWW’Y ’YPṬYSY; i.e., gum; and it is black and laxative

[72] אלווא קַבוּלִינוֹ אלוואי סיטרינום ג׳ מיני׳
’LWW’ QaBWLiYNWo [read: QaBWLiYNYi]; ’LWW’Y SYṬRYNWM; three kinds

[73] איברי ב״א מרוין חם ב״א
’YBRY; German MRWYN; hot in the first degree

[74] אירוקא ב״א אירזול ודומ׳ לחרדל חם ב״ב
’YRWQ’; German ’YRZWL [read: GYRNWL]; it is similar to mustard; [and] hot in the second degree

[75] אלימטי חתים אד׳ תלוי קר ב״א
’LYMṬY ḤTYM ’D’ TLWY; cold in the first degree

[76] איפטיסי ב״א לעבר קרוט חם ב״א
’YPṬYSY; German L‘BR QRWṬ; hot in the first degree

[77] אֵיפִיטִימִי ב״א עשב המשלשל חם ב״א
’eYPiYṬiYMY; German [...]; a laxative; hot in the first degree

[78] אלואנשי ב״א גברנט הזל נושא חם ב״ב
’LW’NŠY [read: ’LW’NYŠ]; German GBRNṬ HZL NWŠ’; hot in the second degree

[79] ארמיפיני אבני׳ הבאי׳ מערמנייא קר ב״ד ומעצר דם
’RMYPYNY [read: ’RMYNYṢY]; stones that come from Armenia; [they are] cold in the fourth degree, and stop a bleeding

[80] אשקולפנדרי ב״א הירצא צונגא קר ב״א
’ŠQWLPNDRY [read: ’ŠQWLPNDRY’]; German HYRṢ’ ṢWNG’; cold in the first degree

[81] אידרי הוא גומ׳ ח״ו ב״ב
’YDRY; i.e., gum; hot and [dry(?)] in the second degree

[82] אומניירישׁ ב״א קפרון חם ולח ב״ב
’WMNYYRYŠ; German QPRWN; hot and moist in the second degree

[83] אורניזא ב״א דורנדִשטֵל קר ולח ב״א י״א בְּרַק וורצא
’WRNYZ’; German DWRNDiŠṬeL; cold and moist in the first degree; some say BəRaQ WWRṢ’

[84] אנטופלי ב״א דיגרוש וויבגעגלכץ חם ב״ב
’NṬWPLY; German DYGRWŠ WWYBG‘GLKṢ [read: WWYSN GLKN]; hot in the second degree

[85] אינטפטי לפיש אבן הנמצ׳ בכבד החזיר
’YNṬPṬY [read: ’YN’PṬY] LPYŠ; a stone that can be found in the liver of a pig

[86] אילימני ב״א ווילדא מגזאמא קר ב״ב
’YLYMNY; German WWYLD’ MGZ’M’; cold in the second degree

3b [87] אגרישטי ב״א שוואנפא מעבר לים
’GRYŠṬY; German ŠWW’NP’; [it can be found] overseas

[88] אשפרמנטום הוא מה שהתרנגול מוציא מפיו
’ŠPRMNṬWM [read: ’ŠPWṬMNṬWM]; i.e., what a cock spits out

[89] אנטימונייא צינא עשא קר ב״ד
’NṬYMWNYY’; German ṢYN’ ‘Š’; cold in the fourth degree

[90] אשטא ב״א ליני ומגדל בפשתן חם ב״ג
’ŠṬ’; German LYNY [read: LYNYN(?)]; it grows in flax; hot in the third degree

[91] איבא ב״א אַבְיוֹן חם ב״ד
’YB’; German ’aBəYWoN; hot in the fourth degree

[92] אפרניקא ב״א לעבור קר ב״ד
’PRNYQ’ [read: ’PRWNY’(?)]; German L‘BWR; cold in the fourth degree

[93] אשטפיזגרא הוא גומ׳ חם ב״ע הרדופני
ʾŠṬPYZGRʾ; i.e., gum; [it is] hot; Hebrew HRDWPNY

[94] אידרא ב״א גונדא רַעַבְא ח״ו ב״ב טוב לקוליקא
ʾYDRʾ; German GWNDʾ RaʿaBəʾ [read: ReʿeBəʾ]; hot and [dry] in the second degree; [it is] good for a colic

[95] איריש ב״א בלַא שווערטל ח״ו ב״ג
ʾYRYŠ; German BLaʾ ŠWWʿRṬL; hot and [dry] in the third degree

[96] אוריגגינו ב״א וינדא חם ב״ב וטוב למי׳ הרעי ונפח
ʾWRYGGYNW [read: ʾWRYGYNW]; German WYNDʾ; hot in the second degree and good for [...] and wind (flatus)

[97] איבולוש ב״א אטיך חם ב״ב
ʾYBWLWŠ; German ʾṬYK; hot in the second degree

[98] אינולא קנפנא ב״א אנלנט חם ולח ב״ג
ʾYNWLʾ QNPNʾ; German ʾNLNṬ [read: ʾLNṬ]; hot and moist in the third degree

[99] איזולא ב״א וולבש מילך ח״ו ב״ג
ʾYZWLʾ; German WWLBŠ MYLK; hot and [dry] in the third degree

[100] אדינטוש ב״א בטוניא קטנ׳ חם ב״א
ʾDYNṬWŠ [read: ʾDYʾNṬWŠ]; German BṬWNYʾ QṬNʾ (minor); hot in the first degree

[101] אמרושקוש ב״א לעבנדיק קאלקא חם ב״ד
ʾMRWŠQWŠ; German LʿBNDYQ QʾLQʾ; hot in the fourth degree

[102] אנטרקליקש ב״א מעלדא חם ב״ב
ʾNṬRQLYQŠ [read: ʾNṬRPLYQŠ]; German MʿLDʾ; hot in the second degree

[103] אמיגְדְלַרוֹם שקדי׳ המרי׳ חמי׳ מתוקי׳ קרי׳
ʾMYGəDəLaRWoM: almonds, bitter, hot, sweet, cold

המרים ב״ט אמיגדלרום אמַרוֹם
the bitter ones [are called] BʾṬ (= be-taytš; i.e., German; h.l., Latin) ʾMYGDLRWM ʾMaRWoM [read: ʾMaRaRWoM]

4a [104] ארבויילקא ב״א נסלין זאמא טוב לאטרופס ומגר׳ השתן פיקקי הנשי׳
'RBWYYLQ'; German NSLYN Z'M'; good for 'ṬRWPS and stimulates urination [...] of women

[105] אנבולא ב״א בערין קרוט חם ויבש ב״ג
'NBWL'; German B'RYN QRWṬ; hot and dry in the third degree

[106] אנאקודי ב״א ווכלדרבר חם ולח
'N'QWDY [read: 'N'QWKY]; German WWKLDRBR; hot and moist

[107] ארנגלושטא ב״א וועגברייד חם ב״ב מחזי׳ הלב והאסטו׳
'RNGLWŠṬ' [read: 'RNGLWŠ']; German WW'GBRYYD; hot in the second degree; it strengthens the heart and the stomach

[108] אישקואיון שחיק ברזל משלשל מאד
'YŠQW'YWN [read: 'YŠQWRYWN]; iron dross; a strong purgative

[109] אנְטֵרַא ב״א רוזן זאמא קר ויבש ב״ב
'NəṬeRa'; German RWZN Z'M'; cold and dry in the second degree

[110] אינטפריום ב״א וולדא זלבא ח״ו ב״ב
'YNṬPRYWM [read: 'YNPṬRYWM]; German WWLD' ZLB'; hot and [dry] in the second degree

[111] ארמוריאצי ב״א ביב׳נעלא
'RMWRY'ṢY; German BYVN'L'

[112] א⟨...⟩יישט ללומן ב״א בֵייְרְא קרוט
'[...]YYŠṬ LLWMN; German BeYYRə' QRWṬ

[113] ארגמין ב״א עברוורין
'RGMYN [read: 'RGMWNY']; German 'BRWWRYN [read: 'BRWWRṢYN]

[114] ארמוניקא ב״א היידריך
'RMWNYQ' [read: 'RMWRYQ']; German HYYDRYK

[115] אינוייר ב״א גונדרום
'YNWYYR; German GWNDRWM

[116] אטרפשטא ב״א הולדר בלומן
'ṬRPŠṬ'; German HWLDR BLWMN

[117] ארקונטילא ב״א קאצין צאגל
'RQWNṬYL'; German Q'ṢYN Ṣ'GL

בית
([Letter] Bet)

[118] בלשמיטא ב״א ברוכא מינצא
BLŠMYṬ'; German BRWK' MYNṢ'

[119] בלשמא ב״א בלשמא חם ב״ב
BLŠM'; German BLŠM'; hot in the second degree

[120] בכלור ב״א לורבר חם ב״ב
BKLWR; German LWRBR; hot in the second degree

[121] בלקשיביזנצי ב״א בישא אוג קר ב״ב 4b
BLQŠYBYZNṢY [read: BLQṬYBYZNṢY']; German BYŠ' [read: PYŠ'] 'WG; cold in the second degree[4]

[122] בולי ארמינסי הוא טיט ארמ⟨נ⟩י קר ב״ד
BWLY 'RMYNSY; i.e., Armenian bole; cold in the fourth degree

[123] בריאוניי ב״א ווילדא קורב⟨...⟩ חם ב״ב
BRY'WNYY; German WWYLD' QWRB⟨...⟩; hot in the second degree

[124] בורטליבי ב״א וורצא קר ב״ה חלוגלות
BWRṬLYBY [read: BWRṬL'KY]; German WWRṢ'; cold; Hebrew ḤLWGLWT [read: ḤLGLGWT]

[125] ביאיין הוא שורש מעבר לים
BY'YYN; this is a root (plant) [that can be found] overseas

4 G. Bos and G. Mensching, "The Black Death in Hebrew Literature: Abraham Ben Solomon Ḥen's *Tractatulus de pestilentia*," *Jewish Studies Quarterly* 18 (2011): 56–57.

[126] בלינקולי ב״א הגון אפלא חם ב״ב
BLYNQWLY; German HGWN [read: HGYN] ʾPLʾ; hot in the second degree

[127] בנדיט מין צוקר קר ב״א
BNDYṬ; a kind of sugar; cold in the first degree

[128] בראנקאורשינא ב״א בערין קלווין חם ב״א
BRʾNQʾWRŠYNʾ [read: BRʾNQʾʾWRŠYNʾ]; German BʿRYN QLWWYN; hot in the first degree

[129] בלושמייש ב״א גרנט אופל בלוט קר ב״א
BLWŠMYYŠ [read: BLWŠṬYYŠ]; German GRNṬ ʾWPL BLWṬ; cold in the first degree

[130] ברדנא ב״א הופא לטיך חם ב״א
BRDNʾ; German HWPʾ LṬYK; hot in the first degree

[131] בדֵלי הוא גומ׳ חם ב״א
BDeLY; i.e., gum; hot in the first degree

[132] בורגין הוא זרע אחד כמו עדשי⟨ם⟩
BWRGYN; i.e., a seed, like lentils

[133] בורייניש הוא בורז בלומין
BWRYYNYŠ [read: BWRGYNYŠ]; i.e., BWRZ BLWMYN

[134][5] בלבטא ב״א אנדורן וטוב לחזה
BLBṬʾ [read: BLWṬʾ]; German ʾNDWRN; good for the chest

[135] ביאטא ב״א איזרין הרץ
BYʾṬʾ; German ʾYZRYN HRṢ

[136] בזילא ב״א מיטר וורץ
BZYLʾ [read: BZYLYʾ]; German MYṬR WWRṢ

5 A marginal entry reads: פולביש אבטיט רצפ׳ פלורוס בילרום בורייניט טימי אניזי ליקוריצי ארמיטרי יישבריש אנ׳ אוק׳ א׳ צניט במשקל בולב.

[137] בזליקוש ב״א מטר קרוט
BZLYQWŠ; German MṬR QRWṬ

[138] בוגלושא ב״א אושון צונגא
BWGLWŠ'; German 'WŠWN [read: 'WQŠYN] ṢWNG'

[139] בריקדיאוש ב״א זב׳נבום
BRYQDY'WŠ; German ZVNBWM

[140] בולוש ב״א בלוטשטיין
BWLWŠ; German BLWṬŠṬYYN

[141] בזילקום ב״א בזילייא
BZYLQWM; German BZYLYY'

[142] ברושקרץ ב״א שטיין ברעכא 5a
BRWŠQRṢ [read: BRWŠQWṢ]; German ŠTYYN BR'K'

אות גימל
(Letter Gimel)

[143] גרופלי ב״א נעלכין חם ב״ג
GRWPLY; German N'LKYN; hot in the third degree

[144] גלגן חם ב״ב
GLGN; hot in the second degree

[145] גלבנום ב״א גלגן חם ב״ב
GLBNWM; German GLGN; hot in the second degree

[146] גרנאני פַּרדִיזִי ב״א פר⟨ד⟩יש קורנר חם ב״ב
GRN'NY [read: GR'NY] PaRDiYZY; German PR[D]YŠ QWRNR; hot in the second degree

[147] גליא מושקדי
GLY' MWŠQDY

[148] גיט ב״א רַאְדָא נמצא בתבוא⟨ות⟩
GYṬ; German Ra'əDə'; it can be found amidst the grain

[149] גוליינא ב״א טושטא
GWLYYN’; German ṬWŠṬ’

[150] גיריט ב״א שווערדל
GYRYṬ [read: GYRWNṬY’]; German ŠWW‘RDL

אות דלת
(Letter Dalet)

[151] דרגנטי ב״א ⟨...⟩ קר ב״ד
DRGNṬY; German [...]; cold in the fourth degree

[152] דאביט ב״א ווילדא ב׳ענכל חם ב״ב
D’BYṬ; German WWYLD’ V‘NKL; hot in the second degree

[153] דעקטילרום ב״א דייטל קערן קר ב״א
D‘QṬYLRWM; German DYYṬL Q‘RN; cold in the first degree

[154] דיאגרידי ב״א הוא שַׁמְנִי חם ב״ג
DY’GRYDY; German ŠaMəNiY; hot in the third degree

[155] דילי הוא ב״א אנדורן חם ב״א
DYLY; German ’NDWRN; hot in the first degree

אות ויו
(Letter Waw)

[156][6] ווילרום ב״א ויאולין קר ב״ב
WWYLRWM [read: WWYWLRWM]; German WY’WLYN; cold in the second degree

[157]ווירגא פשטורי ב״א הירט שטאף
WWYRG’ PŠṬWRY; German HYRT ŠṬ’P

6 Marginal reading: וֵילוּא פֵּנדוֹלא טוב לאבן—WeYLW’ PeNDWoL’; good for stones.

אות טית
(Letter Ṭet)

[158] טטמי משלשל חם
ṬṬMY [read ṬṬM'LY]; it is purging [and] hot

[159] טרבנטינא ב״א לוטר הרצא
ṬRBNṬYN'; German LWṬR HRṢ'

[160] טיטאמי ב״א צוויקלא הוא פרח שחולד׳ מחיי בניה(?)
ṬYṬ'MY [read ṬYṬYM'LY]; German ṢWWYQL'; i.e., a plant that [...]

[161] טפשיאה הוא עשב שעושים בו אחוז׳ עיני׳
ṬPŠY'H; i.e., a plant used for trickery (אחיזת עינים)

אות יוד 5b
(Letter Yod)

[162] יושקיימי ב״א בילזא זאמא קר ב״ד
YWŠQYYMY [read: YWŠQY'MY]; German BYLZ' Z'M'; cold in the fourth degree

[163] יניצייני ב״א אניציון חם ב״ד
YNYṢYYNY; German 'NYṢYWN; hot in the fourth degree

[164] ייט ב״א רַאְדא חם ב״ד
YYṬ; German Ra'əD'; hot in the fourth degree

[165] ייניברי ב״א אינגבר חם ב״ד
YYNYYBRY; German 'YNGBR; hot in the fourth degree

[166] יוניפרי ב״א ווכולטר בֶר חם ב״ב
YWNYPRY; German WWKWLṬR BeR; hot in the second degree

[167] יילצא ב״א טוב וורצא חם ב״ג
YYLṢ'; German ṬWB WWRṢ'; hot in the third degree

אות למד
(Letter Lamed)

[168] לקטוסי ב״א לטיך קר ולח ב״ב
LQṬWSY; German LṬYK; cold and moist in the second degree

[169] ליגנום אלוויש ב״א הימל הולצא חם ב״ב
LYGNWM ʾLWWYŠ; German HYML HWLṢʾ; hot in the second degree

[170] ליגנום צערב״יני ב״א הירץ צונגא חם ב״ב
LYGNWM [read: LYNGWʾ] Ṣʿ RVYNY; German HYRṢ ṢWNGʾ; hot in the second degree

[171] ליגנום אויס ב״א ווגל צונגא חם ב״ב
LYGNWM [read: LYNGWʾ] ʾWYS; German WWGL ṢWNGʾ; hot in the second degree

[172] לוישטיקום ב״א ליבור שטיקול חם ב״א
LWYSṬYQWM; German LYBWR [read: LYBYR] ŠṬYQWL; hot in the first degree

[173] לופינש ב״א ויקא בונא חם ב״ב
LWPYNŠ; German WYQʾ BWNʾ; hot in the second degree

[174] לבריאולא הוא עשב שמגדל עליו שפרינק קורנר
LBRYʾWLʾ; i.e., a plant that grows (on which grow(?)) ŠPRYNQ QWRNR

[175] ליינימש ב״א ציגן ביק חם ב״ד
LYYNYMŠ; German ṢYGN BYQ; hot in the fourth degree

[176] ליטריירום ב״א גולטא עשא חם ויבש ב״ג
LYṬRYYRWM; German GWLṬʾ ʿŠʾ; hot and dry in the third degree

[177] לפיש אמטיטיש ב״א בלוט שטיין קר ב״ד
LPYŠ ʾMṬYṬYŠ; German BLWṬ ŠṬYYN; cold in the fourth degree

[178] לברנום היא גומ׳ חמה
LBRNWM; i.e., gum, hot

[179] לקריצי ב״א לקריץ חם ולח
LQRYṢY; German LQRYṢ; hot and moist

[180] לפיש קלמנריש ב״א קַלְמִין שטיין קר ב״ד
LPYŠ QLMNRYŠ; German QaLəMiYN SṬYYN; cold in the fourth degree

[181] לפיש קלציש ב״א קלקשטיין חם ב״ד 6a
LPYŠ QLṢYŠ; German QLQŠṬYYN; hot in the fourth degree

[182] לפיש לינציש ב״א וולף שטיין
LPYŠ LYNṢYŠ; German WWLP ŠṬYYN

[183] ליטיאמיא ב״א קערש זאמא חם ב״ב
LYṬY'MY'; German Q'RŠ Z'M'; hot in the second degree

[184] לימטוריאורי ב״א גזעגינט גולט חם ב״ד
LYMṬWRY'WRY; German GZ'GYNṬ GWLṬ; hot in the fourth degree

[185] לינטיקולא ב״א לינזין חם ב״ב
LYNṬYQWL'; German LYNZYN; hot in the second degree

[186] לפיש אגפיש הוא השוקף מול השמש
LPYŠ 'GPYŠ; i.e., [the stone] that is transparent in the sun

ונקרא ב״א בריל
and is called in German BRYL

[187] ליברום ונריש ב״א גרוש טישטלא
LYBRWM [read: L'BRWM] WNRYŠ; German GRWŠ ṬYŠṬL'

[188] לקטידא ב״א שפנא וורץ
LQṬYD' [read: LQṬYRYD']; German ŠPN' [read: ŠPYN'] WWRṢ

[189] לילפנוש ב״א זלבייא
LYLPNWŠ [read: LYLPGWŠ]; German ZLBYY'

[190] לאבדנום הוא גומ׳ מעבר לים חם ולח ב״א
L'BDNWM; i.e., gum [that can be found] overseas; it is hot and moist in the first degree

[191] ליליום ב״א לוליין חם ולח בראשו׳
LYLYWM; German LWLYYN [read: LYLYYN]; hot and moist in the first degree

[192] לפיש לזולי הוא אבן לזור קר ויבש
LPYŠ LZWLY; i.e., the stone [called] LZWR; cold and dry

[193] ליניש ב״א לינא חם ולח
LYNYŠ; German LYN'; hot and moist

[194] ליציאוש חם ב״ד ויבש בשני המי׳ טובי׳ לעיני׳
LYṢY'WŠ [read: LYṢY'WM]; hot in the fourth degree and dry in the second degree; the juice is good for the eyes

[195] לאפציום ב״א קלעטין קרוטא חם ויבש
L'PṢYWM; German QL'ṬYN QRWṬ'; hot and dry

[196] לבג׳ ונמצא גדול וקטן
LBĞ; there is a large and small variety

[197] לאורוש ב״א לורברן בום חם ויבש
L'WRWŠ; German LWRBRN BWM; hot and dry

[198] לינטיקוש ב״א ליאיזין חם ויבש
LYNṬYQWŠ [read: LYNṬYŠQWŠ]; German LY'YZYN; hot and dry

[199] לוריאולא ב״א שפרינק קורנר וב״ט
LWWRY'WL'; German ŠPRYNQ QWRNR [...](?)

[200] לקטיפוציא ונותן חלב ח״ו ב״ג
LQṬYPWṢY'; it gives milk; it is hot and [...] in the third degree

6b [201] לפיש ארמיניקוש הוא אבן מארמֶנְייא
LPYŠ 'RMYNYQWŠ; i.e., a stone from Armenia

[202] לפיש פיריציש ב״א ב׳ור שטיין
LPYŠ PYRYṢYŠ; German VWWR ŠṬYYN

אות מם
(Letter Mem)

[203] משטיסי ב״א משטיק חם ב״ב
MŠTYSY [read: MŠTYSYŠ]; German MŠṬYQ; hot in the second degree

[204] מיליום שוליש ב״א שטיין ברעכא חם ב״ב
MYLYWM ŠWLYŠ; German ŠṬYYN BR‘K’; hot in the second degree

[205] מנדרגורא ב״א אלרונא קר ב״ד
MNDRGWR’; German ’LRWN’; cold in the fourth degree

[206] מְרְגַרטרום ב״א פערלין חם ב״ב
MRəGaRṬRWM [read: MRəGaRṬ’RWM]; German P‘RLYN; hot in the second degree

[207] מאציש ב״א מושקדן בלומן חם ב״ב
M’ṢYŠ; German MWŠQDN BLWMN; hot in the second degree

[208] מאַרְטְרִי ב״א וונכל זאמא חם ב״ב
M’aRəṬəRiY; German WWNKL Z’M’; hot in the second degree

[209] מרוֹבְיוֹ ב״א אנדורן חם ב״ב
MRWoBəYWo [read: MRWoBiYWuM]; German ’NDWRN; hot in the second degree

[210] מומי ב״א טודן ב׳לייש חם ב״ב
MWMY [read: MWMY’]; German ṬWDN VLYYŠ; hot in the second degree

[211] מוי ב״א בלדריון קר ב״א
MWY; German BLDRYWN; cold in the first degree

[212] מילינצי ב״א זומר אופל חם ב״ב
MYLYNṢY; German ZWMR ’WPL; hot in the second degree

[213] מושקי ב״א ביזמא חם ב״ב
MWŠQY; German BYZM’; hot in the second degree

[214] מינרוניקא ב״א ווילדא פטרסליא חם ב״ב
MYNRWNYQ’; German WWYLD’ PṬRSLY’; hot in the second degree

[215] מלילוטום ב״א קונגש קרונא
MLYLWṬWM; German QWNGŠ QRWN’

[216] מייטילי ב״א היידלבר קר ב״ד
MYYṬYLY [read: MYRṬYLY]; German HYYDLBR; cold in the fourth degree

[217] מואמן ב״א בראנבר קר ב״א
MW'MN [read: MWRWM]; German BR'NBR; cold in the first degree

[218] מוראש ב״א מולבר קר ב״ב
MWR'Š [read: MWR']; German MWLBR; cold in the second degree

[219] מלוניש ב״א מילדא קר ב״ב
MLWNYŠ; German MYLD'; cold in the second degree

[220] מלוא ב״א פאפל קר ולח ב״א
MLW'; German P'PL; cold and moist in the first degree

ביש מלוא ב״א איבש קר ולח ב״ב
BYŠ MLW'; German 'YBŠ; cold and moist in the second degree

7a[7] [221] מילשא היא גומ׳ והוא זבל שטן
MYLŠ'; i.e., gum, i.e., "devil's dung"

[222] מריני ב״א במעקן
MRYNY; German BM'QN

[223] מורביצי ב״א ברונבר
MWRBYṢY [read: MWRWM RBYSY]; German BRWNBR

[224] מלילוזא ב״א מֵטְרְא
MLYLWZ' [read: MLYZ']; German MeṬəRə'

[225] מורֵילא ב״א נהשטא
MWReYL'; German NHŠṬ' [read: NHṬŠṬ']

[226] מומינא ב״א זיילא וורץ
MWMYN' [read: MYMYṬ']; German ZYYL' WWRṢ

7 The top margin of fol. 7a has the entry: מלילוטוס מרכך (melilot has a softening (laxative) effect).

[227] ממכרוזייא ב״א גרווא
MMKRWZYY'; German GRWW'

[228] מארטרום ב״א וועגכל
M'RṬRWM; German WW'NKL

[229] מושקוקאן ב״א קולא זאן
MWŠQWQ'N; German QWL' Z'N

[230] מרבלני סיטריני אינדי בִּילַרֵיצֵיא אימליסי קיבולי כולם מין אחד הוא ונכנסי׳ בלקשטין
MRBLNY SYṬRYNY; 'YNDY; BiYLaReYṢeY'; 'YMLYSY; QYBWLY; all of them are of one kind and enter into (are used for) LQŠṬYN [read: LQŠYRN]

[231] מילסא הוא גומ׳ מרצי הוא בונעקין
MYLS'; i.e., gum; MRṢY; i.e., BWN'QYN

[232] מנא ב״א הימלש בראט
MN'; German HYMLŠ BR'Ṭ

אות נון
(Letter Nun)

[233] ניילַא ב״א ראדין חם ב״ב
NYYLa'; German R'DYN; hot in the second degree

[234] ניפרי ב״א קלי בלומין
NYPRY; German QLY BLWMYN

[235] נוציש בומי ב״א וויליט נוס
NWṢYŠ BWMY; German WWYLYṬ NWS

[236] נוציש מושקדי ב״א מושקט נושא חם ב״ב
NWṢYŠ MWŠQDY; German MWŠQṬ NWŠ'; hot in the second degree

[237] נרְדוֹשְׁטַצְיוֹס אונ׳ נרדוש ⟨ו⟩אנדיקא הוא שפיק נרדי
NRəDWoŠəṬaṢəYWoS and NRDWŠ 'NDYQ'; i.e., ŠPYQ [read: ŠPYQ'] NRDY

[238] נרדוש צלטיקא הוא שפיק סלטיקא
NRDWŠ ṢLṬYQ'; i.e., ŠPYQ [read: ŠPYQ'] SLṬYQ'

[239] נַפיאָה ב״א זענף זאמא
NaPY'aH [read: NaPY]; German Z'NP Z'M'

[240] נרְדִלְיוֹן הוא שמן נרדי
NRəDiLəYWoN; i.e., nard oil

7b [241] נֶפְטַא ב״א מינטא
NePəṬa'; German MYNṬ'

[242] נוקש מִרְאִשְׁטִיקָא ב״א מושקט נושא
NWQŠ MiRə'iŠəṬiYQa'; German MWŠQṬ NWŠ'

[243] נוקש פוֹנְטִיקָא ב״א הזל נושא
NWQŠ PWoNəṬiYQa'; German HZL NWŠ'

אות סמך
(Letter Samekh)

[244] סטורקש הוא ג׳ מיני גומא האחד נקר׳ שטורק קלמיטי והב׳ רוביא והוא הפסולת מן הראשו׳ והג׳ שטורק קומפיטא והוא הפסול׳ מן קוֹזִימְבֵּרוֹם
SṬWRQŠ; i.e., three kinds of gum; the first is called ŠṬWRQ [read: SṬWRQŠ] QLMYṬY; the second RWBY'; i.e., the dregs of the first; the third is ŠṬWRQ [read: SṬWRQŠ] QWMPYṬ' and this is the dregs of QWoZiYMəBeRWoM [read: QWoZiYMəBeRWuM]

[245] סטורציש קלמנטא ב״א שטיק נרדי חם ב״ב
SṬWRṢYŠ QLMNṬ'; German ŠṬYQ NRDY; hot in the second degree

[246] סליונצי ב״א ווילדא קומא חם ב״ב
SLYWNṢY; German WWYLD' QWM'; hot in the second degree

[247] סילי מונטעני ב״א גרושא זאמא
SYLY MWNṬ'NY; German GRWŠ' Z'M'

[248] סשקְטְפי(?) ב״א עבור וורצא
SŠQəṬəPY(?); German 'BWR [read: 'BYR] WWRṢ'

[249] סולפר ב״א שוועבל חם ב״א
SWLPR; German ŠWW'BL; hot in the first degree

[250] ספיסי ב״א ווילדא שפיק חם ב״ב
SPYSY; German WWYLD' ŠPYQ; hot in the second degree

[251] שילו בלשמי הוא העץ ח׳ ב״ב
ŠYLW BLŠMY; this is the tree; hot in the second degree

[252] שלויאה ב״א זֵלְבְא ח׳ ב״ב
ŠLWY'H; German ZeLəBə'; hot in the second degree

[253] שיטרינום הוא מגדל באילן ח׳ ב״ב
ŠYṬRYNWM; it grows on a tree; hot in the second degree

[254] סנפוצי ב״א הולנדר חם ב״ב
SNPWṢY [read: SNBWṢY]; German HWLNDR; hot in the second degree

[255] סנְבוֹקוֹש גם הולנדר והוא פורח בשנ׳ י״ב מאות׳ פרחי׳ מתקני׳ שמן שַׁנְבוֹצִינוֹם
SNəBWoQWoŠ [read: SNəBWoQWuŠ]; also [called] HWLNDR; it gets flowers twelve times a year; from these flowers they make ŠaNəBWoṢiYNWoM [read: ŠaNəBWoṢiYNWuM] oil

[256] סוליני ב״א ליני זאמא חם ב״א 8a[8]
SWLYNY [read: SMN LYNY]; German LYNY Z'M'; hot in the first degree

[257] סטיפיטרקרום הוא שורש טחול
SṬYPYṬRQRWM; i.e., the "root of the spleen"

[258] סבינה ב״א זאב״ין בום חם ב״ב
SBYN'; German Z'VYN BWM; hot in the second degree

[259] סטורציום ב״א ווילדא קול
SṬWRṢYWM; German WWYLD' QWL

---

8 Fol. 8a has a marginal entry of a recipe for blackening a person in the bathhouse (?): להשחיר אדם במרחץ: קח עפר גלש וקופרוזא והשלך עליו ולא יתלבן רק ברוב מים חמין ואם תשים העפר במי׳ קרים ידיו בו יושחרו.

[260] סיטרולי ב״א זומר אופל חם ב״ב
SYṬRWLY; German ZWMR 'WPL; hot in the second degree

[261] סנגווי דרכוניש הוא מוהל של עשב ואיננו דם תנין
SNGWWY [read: SNGWWYŠ] DRKWNYŠ; that is the juice of plants and it is not DM TNYN (dragon's blood; i.e., resin of the Socotra dragontree [*Dracaena cinnabari* Balf. f.]).

[262] סילירום ב״א אברוש חם ב״ד
SYLYRWM; German 'BRWŠ; hot in the fourth degree

[263] סליש קמוני מלח שלנו
SLYŠ QMWNY [read: QMWNYŠ]; our salt (common salt)

[264] שלניטרי הוא מלח אחר יתקנו ממנו אש זרה
ŠLNYṬRY; this is another [kind of] salt; 'Š ZRH (artificial fire; i.e., saltpeter) is made from it

[265] סנוגריקום ב״א קריש הווא
SNWGRYQWM [read: PNWGRYQWM]; German QRYŠ HWW'

[266] סזוִילַא ב״א מר צוויבול
SZWiYLa' [read: SQWiYLa']; German MR ṢWWYBWL [read: ṢWWYBYL]

[267] סומק הוא זרע שחור קר ב״ב ומעצר
SWMQ; it is a black seed; cold in the second degree and astringent

[268] ספודיום ב״א גברנט חלפין בַיין וי״א הוא שורש שרוף כמו גלגן שמן בוֹנְבַצִיש ב״א בוואמא וולא זאמא
SPWDYWM; German GBRNṬ ḤLPYN [read: HLPYN] BaYYN; some say that it is a burnt root; like GLGN; ŠMN BWoNəBaṢiYŠ; German BWW'M' [read: B'WWM] WWL' Z'M'

[269] סוקוש לקרוצי הוא מוהל שלו
SWQWŠ LQRWṢY [read: LQRYṢY]; i.e., its juice

[270] סרפינא הוא גומ׳ ויש קור׳ סאגפינום
SRPYN' [read: SRPYNWM]; i.e., gum; some call [it] S'GPYNWM

[271] סרקקולא הוא גומ׳ חם שם אח׳ גלוטינום
SRQQWL’; i.e., gum; hot; another name: GLWṬYNWM

[272] סינאופי ב״א זענף חם ב״ב
SYN’WPY [read: SYN’PY]; German Z‘NP; hot in the second degree

[273] סינמומי הוא קנלא ב״א 8b
SYNMWMY; i.e., QNL’ in German

[274] שֶׁפַּרְווִיף ב״א הושא ווירצא קר ב״ד
ŠePaRəWWYP [read: ŠeMPaRəWWYPWM]; German HWŠ’ [read: HWŠ] WWYRṢ’; cold in the fourth degree

[275] שולְטְרוֹ ב״א נהטא שאדא קר ב״ד
ŠWLəṬəRWo; German NHṬ’ Š’D’; cold in the fourth degree

[276] שקווינגטום פַּלֵיאָה קַמַלַרוֹם ב״א מין קש
ŠQWWYNNṬWM; PaLeY’aH QaMaLaRWoM [read: QaMaLaRWuM] in German; [Hebrew] a kind of straw

[277] שיני הם עלים של אילן
ŠYNY; i.e., the leaves of a tree

[278] שַקְשִיפְּרְיַיא ב״א שטיין ברעכא
ŠaQəŠiYPəRəYYa’; German ŠṬYYN BR‘K’

[279] שִינַנוּם פֶּטַרְסְלִינוּם אגרישטי ב״א ווילדא פטרסיליא
ŠYiNaNWM; PeṬaRəSəLiYNWM ’GRYŠṬY; German WWYLD’ PṬRSYLY’

[280] שנדרקא אאורי פִּיקְמַנְטוֹם רוביום
ŠNDRQ’; ’’WRY PiYQəMaNəṬWoM [read: PiYQəMaNəṬWuM] RWBYWM

[281] שולְפֵּנְדִירְיַא לינגנום צֵירְוֶנַא ב״א הירץ צונגא
ŠWLəPeNəDYRəYa’ [read: ŠQWLəPeNəDYRəYa’]; LYNGNWM [read: LYNGW’] ṢeYRəWeNa’; German HYRṢ ṢWNG’

[282] שמִירְיוש ביטוניקא ב״א בטונייא
ŠMiYRəYWŠ; BYṬWNYQ’; German BṬWNYY’

אות עין
(Letter Ayin)

[283] ענמברא י״א ביבא מרג הנקר׳ בלייניי וי״א שנולד בקרקע הים חם ויבש ב״ב
'NMBR' [read: 'MBR']; some say: BYB' MRG that is called BLYYNYY and others say that it hails from the bottom of the sea; hot and dry in the second degree

אות פה
(Letter Pe)

[284] פנאמי פיאניש ב״א וילדא רוטא חם ב״ב
PN'MY [delete] PY'NYŠ [read: PG'NY]; German WYLD' RWṬ'; hot in the second degree

[285] פולי ב״א נעגלכין בְלֵטֶר חם ב״ב
PWLY [read: PWLYY]; German N'GLKYN BəLeṬeR; hot in the second degree

[286] פיפר לוניי ב״א לאנגא פעפר חם ב״ג
PYPR LWNYY; German L'NG' P'PR; hot in the third degree

[287] פטרסליני ב״א פטרסיליא חם ב״ב
PṬRSLYNY; German PṬRSYLY'; hot in the second degree

[288] פיטיר ב״א בחט רום חם ב״ב
PYṬYR [read: PYRYṬRWM]; German BḤṬ RWM [read: BRḤṬRM]; hot in the second degree

[289] פיגמי ב״א שטאבאווירצא חם ב״ג
PYGMY [read: PYGNY]; German ŠṬ'B' WWYRṢ'; hot in the third degree

9a [290] פליי ב״א גרווא חם ב״ב
PLYY [read: PLYY']; German GRWW'; hot in the second degree

[291] פראשִי ב״א אנדיק לבן חם ב״ב
PR'ŠiY [read: PR'ŠiYY]; German white 'NDYQ [read: 'NDWRN]; hot in the second degree

[292] פניקולי ב״א וועגכל חם ב״ב
PNYQWLY; German WWʿNKL; hot in the second degree

[293] פרלי ב״א בריל הוא קרישטל קר ב״ד
PRLY; German BRYL; i.e., QRYŠṬL; cold in the fourth degree

[294] פוליטריקום ב״א ניזא וורצא חם ב״ד
PWLYṬRYQWM; German NYZ' WWRṢ'; hot in the fourth degree

[295] פולי ציטריני ב״א געלא ליליין חם ב״ב
PWLY [read: PWLYY] ṢYṬRYNY; German GʿL' LYLYYN; hot in the second degree

[296] פטר אלי ב״א אליי מֵרומְא חם ב״ב
PṬR 'LY [read: PṬR'LYY]; German 'LYY from Rome; hot in the second degree

[297] פוי ב״א באלדריון חם ב״ב
PWY [read: PW]; German B'LDRYWN; hot in the second degree

[298] פיאוניש ב״א בנוניון קורנר חם ב״ב
PY'WNYŠ [read: PY'WNY']; German BNWNYYWN [read: BGWNYYWN] QWRNR; hot in the second degree

[299] פינים ב״א טאנאפל חם ב״ב
PYNYM [read: PYNWM]; German Ṭ'N'PL; hot in the second degree

[300] פרוניש ב״א פרומין קר ב״ב
PRWNYŠ [read: PRWNWM]; German PRWMYN; cold in the second degree

[301] פייא נאבליש ב״א פעך ב׳ון שיפאן חם ב״ב
PYY' [read: PYQŠ] N'BLYŠ; German PʿK VWN ŠYP'N; hot in the second degree

[302] פולפודיום ב״א הומול חם ב״ד
PWLPWDYWM; German HWMWL; hot in the fourth degree

[303] פינדאני ב״א ווילד וועגכל
PYND'NY [read: PWQD'NY]; German WWYLD WWʿNKL

[304] פומא סיטריני הוא אתרוג יש בו ג׳ טבעי׳ הקליפ׳ חם והבשר קר
PWM’ [read: PWMY] SYṬRYNY; i.e., citron; it has three natures; the peel is hot [read: cold] and the flesh is cold [read: hot]

[305] פומטערא פְלאמֵנוש ב״א טובן קרופא חם בג׳
PWMṬ‘R’ [read: PWMYṬ‘R’]; PəL’MeNWŠ; German ṬWBN QRWP’ [read: QRWP]; hot in the third degree

[306] פומטערא ב״א ערטא רוטא חם ב״ג
PWMṬ‘R’ [read: PWMYṬ‘R’]; German ‘RṬ’ [read: ‘RṬ] RWṬ’; hot in the third degree

[307] פילוזילא ב״א מוזא אורא חם ב״ב
PYLWZYL’; German MWZ’ ’WR’; hot in the second degree

[308] פְלַמולַא הוא עשב ח״ו ב״ד והלועס בפיו ישרף באש בלשון
PəLaMWLa’; it is a herb that is hot and [dry] in the fourth degree; if someone chews it in his mouth, his tongue will be burned

9b [309] פיזגרא ב״א ציזרין חם ב״ד
PYZGR’ [read: ŠṬPYZGR’]; German ṢYZRYN; hot in the fourth degree

[310] פובטגיש ב״א וויגריך חם ב״א
PWBṬGYŠ [read: PLNṬGYNYŠ]; German WWYGRYK; hot in the first degree

[311] פישטצירום ב״א נושא הזל חם ב״ב
PYŠṬṢYRWM; German NWŠ’ HZL; hot in the second degree

[312] פיניארום ב״א וועלשא נושא חם ב״ב
PYNY’RWM; German WW‘LŠ’ NWŠ’; hot in the second degree

[313] פוליון ב״א פוליי חם ב״ב
PWLYWN [read: PWLYWM]; German PWLYY; hot in the second degree

[314] פריטיקום ב״א בחטרום
PRYṬYQWM [read: PYRYṬYQWM]; German BḤṬRWM [read: BRḤṬRM]

[315] פיריטרטריא ב״א נהט אונ׳ טאק הם ב׳ עשבי׳
PYRYṬRṬRY’ [read: PYRYṬRY’]; German NHṬ ’WN T’Q; these are two herbs

[316] פורטישקילא ב״א גרנזינק
PWRṬYŠQYL’ [read: PWRṬNṬYL’]; German GRNZYNQ

[317] פלוטרקום ב״א שטיין ברעכא
PLWṬRQWM [read: PWLṬRYQWM]; German ŠṬYYN BR‘K’

[318] פששינק ב״א מורכן
PŠŠYNQ [read: PŠṬYNQ’]; German MWRKN

[319] פראולי ב״א אגרמונייא
PR’WLY; German ’GRMWNYY’ [read: ’GRMWND’]

[320] פופיפיריש ב״א ביזון
PWPYPYRYŠ [read: PWPYRWŠ]; German BYZWN

[321] פיגנוא ב״א וולא רוטן
PYGNW’ [read: PYGNWM]; German WWL’ [read: WWLD] RWṬN

[322] פיפפניל ב״א ביב׳נעלא
PYPPNYL [read: PYPYNYL’]; German BYVN‘L’

[323] פצינמומי ב״א צינמין חם
PṢYNMWMY [read: ṢYNMWMY]; German ṢYNMYN; hot

אות צדי
(Letter Ṣade)

[324] צדוורי ב״א צדוון חם ב״ב
ṢDWWRY; German ṢDWWN; hot in the second degree

[325] ציקלמין ב״א שווינש ברוט
ṢYQLMYN; German ŠWWYNŠ BRWṬ

[326] צנטרירום ב״א קוודין קערנא
ṢNṬRYRWM; German QWWDYN Q‘RN’

[327] ציפרי ב״א ווילדא גלגן חם ב״ב
ṢYPRY; German WWYLD’ GLGN; hot in the second degree

10a [328] ציטרולי ב״א ערדא אפלא קר ב״ב
ṢYṬRWLY; German ‘RD’ ’PL’; cold in the second degree

[329] צנטווריאה יש ב׳ מיני׳ גדול וקטן וקורי׳ הגוי (= הגד׳(?)) פשתן של ⟨...⟩
ṢNṬWWRY’H; there are two varieties: large and small; the large(?) one is called “flax of [...]”

[330] צירוסא ב״א בלי עשא
ṢYRWS’; German BLY ‘Š’

[331] ציפי ב״א צוויבולן
ṢYPY; German ṢWWYBWLN

[332] צישושלא ב״א עַרְבֵר
ṢYŠWŠL’; German ‘aRəBeR

[333] צירי פוליום ב״א קירבל
ṢYRY PWLYWM; German QYRBL

[334] ציטונום ב״א קומל
ṢYṬWNWM; German QWML

[335] צילי רוניא ב״א שֵׁלא וורץ
ṢYLY RWNY’ [read: ṢYLYDWNY’]; German ŠeL’ [read: ŠeL] WWRṢ

[336] צירני ב״א ווילדא קומל
ṢYRNY; German WWYLD’ QWML

[337] ציקולמא ב״א אִידִין אֵפל
ṢYQWLM’; German ’iYDiYN ’ePL

[338] צימברי ⟨...⟩ שנמבוקי ב״א הולנדר
ṢYMBRY [...] ŠNMBWQY [read: ŠMBWQY]; German HWLNDR

[339] ציקרי ב״א ווענא וויזא
ṢYQRY; German WW‘G’ WWYZ’

קוף
([Letter] Qof)

[340] קרפו בלשמי ב״א הולץ ב׳ון בלשו קר ולח וי״א חם ב״ב
QRPW BLŠMY; German HWLṢ VWN BLŠW [read: BLŠM]; cold and moist; some say: hot in the second degree

[341] קשייא ליגני ב״א ווילדא צינמין
QŠYY' LYGNY [read: QŠYY' LYGNY']; German WWYLD' ṢYNMYN

[342] קושטי ב״א ווילדא צידוון וי״א כי הוא ריברבא חם ב״ב
QWŠṬY [read: QWŠQWṬ']; German WWYLD' ṢYDWWN; some say that it is RYBRB'; hot in the second degree

[343] קלמנטא ב״א שפיק נֵרְדא ח׳ ב״ב 10b
QLMNṬ'; German ŠPYQ NaRəD'; hot in the second degree

[344] קרדמומי חם ב״ב
QRDMWMY; hot in the second degree

[345] קשטורייא ב״א ביבר געיילא ח׳ ב״ג
QŠṬWRYY' [read: QŠṬWRYY]; German BYBR G'YYL'; hot in the third degree

[346] קמרדי ב״א גמרדי ח׳ ב״ב
QMRDY [read: QMDRYWŠ]; German GMRDY [read: GMNDR]; hot in the second degree

[347] קלמי ארמטיסי ב״א מר הֶלמא בא מרומני חם ב״ב
QLMY 'RMṬYSY; German MR HeLM' [read: HeLM] that hails from Romania(?); hot in the second degree

[348] קרווי ב״א וושא קומל חם ב״ב
QRWWY; German WWŠ' QWML; hot in the second degree

[349] קרוצי ב״א גרטון זפרון ח׳ ב״ב
QRWṢY; German GRṬWN [read: GRṬYN] ZPRWN; hot in the second degree

[350] קשיא פישטל קר במעל׳ ראשונ׳
QSY’ PYŠṬL [read: PYŠṬL’]; cold in the first degree

[351] קנמפרי קר ב״ד
QNMPRY [read: QNPRY]; cold in the fourth degree

[352] קוריצי נידי ב״א שֶלוטא ב׳ון שפינל שם ח׳ ב״ב
QWRYṢY [read. QWRYṢYY] NYDY; German ŠeLWṬ’ VWN ŠPYNL ŠM; hot in the second degree

[353] קריטיסי ב״א ב׳יגין ח׳ ב״א
QRYṬYSY; German VYGYN; hot in the first degree

[354] קולקוונטדי ב״א מר אופל והם לקשטיף ח׳ ב״ב
QWLQWWNṬDY [read: QWLQWYNṬDYŠ]; German MR ’WPL and they are LQŠṬYP; hot in the second degree

[355] קוקנידי ב״א שפריקא וורצא זאמא ח׳ ב״ג
QWQNYDY; German ŠPRYQ’ WWRṢ’ [read: WWRṢ] Z’M’; hot in the third degree

[356] קוקורביט ב״א קורבש קר ב״א
QWQWRBYṬ [read: QWQWRBYṬ’]; German QWRBŠ [read: QWRBYŠ]; cold in the first degree

[357] קלופוניא ב״א קרישפך ח׳ ב״ב
QLWPWNY’; German QRYŠPK; hot in the second degree

[358] קאממילא חם ב״ב
Q’MMYL’; hot in the second degree

[359] קורנו ליאוניש בשר אריה ח׳ ב״ב
QWRNW LY’WNYŠ; lion’s flesh; hot in the second degree

11a [360] קושקוטי ב״א משי שרף(?) ח׳ ב״ב
QWŠQWṬY; German MŠY ŠRP(?); hot in the second degree

[361] קפריש ב״א רוטא קולא גרוש
QPRYŠ [read: QPRWŠ]; German RWṬ’ QWL’ GRWŠ

Entries 362–375 are partly illegible due to severe staining

[362] קמיפטיאוש גמנדרי די גרושא ח׳ ב״ב
QMYPṬY'WŠ; GMNDRY DY GRWŠ'; hot in the second degree

[363] קוביביש ⟨...⟩
QWBYBYŠ [...]

[364] קוריינדרי ⟨...⟩
QWRYYNDRY [...]

[365] קטפוצייא ב״א ש⟨פריי⟩נך(?) וורצא(?)
QTPWṢYY'; German Š[PRYY]NK(?) WWRṢ'(?) [read: WWRṢ]

[366] קפליא ונרוש(?) ב״א שיינא(?)
QPLY' WNRWŠ(?) [read: QPLY WNRYŠ]; German ŠYYN'(?) [read: ŠṬYYN' [RWṬ(?)]

[367] קונסולדא ⟨...⟩ ג׳ מיני׳(?) ב״א וולא(?) די גרושא(?)
QWNSWLD' [read: QWNSWLYD'] [...]; three species(?); German WWL'(?) [read: WWL] DY GRWŠ'(?)

[368] קרבוסנבנדיקט(?) ב״א שטורצא וורצא
QRBWSNBNDYQṬ(?) [read: QRDWS BNDYQṬWŠ]; German ŠṬWRṢ' WWRṢ'

[369] קרקולא ב״א דרוש וורצא
QRQWL' [read: QRSWL']; German DRWŠ WWRṢ'

[370] קיטלא בישטולאה(?) ב״א הונדש(?) וורצא בלומין
QYṬL' BYŠṬWL'H(?) [read: QWṬWL' PYṬYD']; German HWNDŠ (?) WWRṢ' BLWMYN

[371] קמלוש ב״א הומש(?) צדוון(?)
QMLWŠ; German HWMŠ(?) [read: HWNDŠ(?)] ṢDWWN(?)

[372] קממולא ב״א מיידא בלומין
QMMWL' [read: QMMYL']; German MYYD' [read: MYY] BLWMYN

[373] קוקריאון ב״א מאיניו(?)
QWQRY'WN; German M'YNYW(?)

[374] קולמבדיא ב״א שטרן וורצא
QWLMBDY' [read: QWLMBRY']; German ŠṬRN WWRṢ'

[375] קלינדולא ב״א רינגל קרוט
QLYNDWL'; German RYNGL QRWṬ

[376] קלמנטום ב״א שטיינא מינצא
QLMNṬWM; German ŠṬYYN' MYNṢ'

[377] קרדניאום ב״א ווילדא קרעש
QRDNY'WM [read: QRDMWNY'WM]; German WWYLD' QR'Š

[378] קונקונתום ב״א איידרמנט ח׳ ב״ג
QWNQWNTWM [read: QLQNTWM]; German 'YYDRMNṬ [read: 'TRMNṬ]; hot in the third degree

11b **ריש**

([Letter] Resh)

[379] ריבארבא ב״א ⟨...⟩
RYB'RB'; German [...]

[380] רפונטקום ב״א וורצלא ב׳ון טורקייא ח׳ ב״ב ודומה לריברבא
RPWNṬQWM; German WWRṢL' VWN ṬWRQYY'; hot in the second degree and similar to RYBRB'

[381] רפאני ב״א מר רטיך ח׳ ב״ג
RP'NY; German MR RṬYK; hot in the third degree

Edition of Glossary 2 (fols. 11b–17b)

אלפא בית אחר 11b

(Another alphabet[ical list])

[1] אַרְמַרִיאַקוֹס ג׳ שמות יש לו א׳ שַׁנְשׁוּקוּשׁ ב׳ מיארנא ג׳ אוליבריום ד׳ פערשא הו׳ מארצין

’aRəMaRiY’aQWoS; it has three (?) names: (1) ŠaNəŠWuQWŠ; (2) MY’RN’; (3) ’WLYBRYWM; (4) P‘RŠ’; i.e., M’RṢYN

[2] אדרשקא א׳ אליברוס אלבוש ב״א ניזיא וורצין

’DRŠQ’ [or] ’LYBRWS ’LBWŠ; German NYZY’ WWRṢYN

[3] אמֶנְטֵילַא ב״א בלדיריון אונ׳ טִיטְיַרְקְא ו׳ שמות יש לו פוֹנְטִילַא טוֹרמַנְטִילַא מאנטילא פ׳ו ווילירינא

’MeNəṬeYLa’; German BLDYRYWN and ṬiYṬəYaRəQə’ [read: ṬYRY’Q’]; it has six names: PWoNəṬiYLa’ [read: PWṬNṬYL’]; ṬWoRMaNəṬYLa’; M’NṬYL’; FW; WWYLYRYN’ [read: WWYLYRY’N’] [...]

[4] אלִימְפִיַאדוס הם שורש אותו עשב וזרע שלו ב״ט קוֹקנדיון ב״א צידלבשט

’LiMəPiYa’DWS; i.e., the root and seed of that plant; Latin QWoQNDYWN; German ṢYDLBŠṬ

[5] אפ׳ודִילִי ב״א ווילדא לוך ג׳ שמו׳ י״ל אַלְבוציום צנטום קאפיטא

’FWDiYLiY; German WWYLD’ LWK; it has three names: ’aLəBWṢYWM; ṢNṬWM Q’PYṬ’

[6] אַגריקום ב״א טאנין שומעין

’aGRYQWM; German Ṭ’NYN ŠWM‘YN

[7] אַריסטלוניי רטונדא ב״א הולא ווירצא זינוול

’aRYSṬLWNYY RṬWND’; German HWL’ WWYRṢ’ ZYNWWL

[8] אַרְטִימֵשׁ קֵפִנֵלִין ב״א קאמילא בלומין

’aRəṬiYMeŠ; QePiNeLiYN; German Q’MYL’ BLWMYN

[9] אַמֵאוש ב״א בזיליין זאמא גשיל נֵאִיטא צִינִימֵלַא

’aMc’WŠ; German BZYLYYN Z’M’; GŠYL Ne’iYṬ’; ṢiYNiYMeLa’

 | DOI:10.1163/9789004459380_004

12a [10] אננייא א׳ ב׳ פפב׳ריש רוביום ב״א רוט מגזאמא פפבריש אלבי ב״א וויש מגזא׳ ב״ט קוֹדְיוֹן מיקא
'NNYY' [read: 'NMWN'] [two species] PPVRYŠ RWBYWM; German RWṬ MGZ'M'; PPBRYŠ 'LBY; German WWYŠ MGZ''; Latin QWoDəYWoN; MYQ'

[11] ארנגלוסא ב״א שפִּייגץ(?) ווגריך ושיל
'RNGLWS'; German ŠPiYYGṢ(?) [read: ŠPiYṢ] WWGRYK; WŠYL

[12] אדיאנטוש ב״ט קפילי ונריִש ב״א ווידר טאט
'DY'NṬWŠ; Latin QPYLY WNRYiš; German WWYDR Ṭ'Ṭ

[13] איריש ב״א שווערטלין וייש בלווין ליליין
'YRYŠ; German ŠWW'RṬLYN; WYYŠ BLWWYN; LYLYYN

[14] אריאוש יש לו פרחים לבנים
'RY'WŠ; it has white flowers

[15] אקורוש גלדיילוש יש להם געלא בלומ׳
'QWRWŠ; GLDYYLWŠ [read: GLDYWLWŠ]; they have G'L' BLWM' (yellow flowers)

[16] אלילויא ב״א גוקש לוך
'LYLWY'; German GWQŠ LWK

[17] אילַקְטרִיום הוא מוקל מן קשואי׳ ווילדא
'YLaQəṬRiYWM; i.e., juice from WWYLD' (wild) cucumbers

[18] אריצינא(?) הוא עשב ששמו שפְּריש
'RYṢYN'(?); i.e., a plant called ŠPəRYŠ

[19] אירבא פּוֹלוניִש הוא ע׳ וזרע שלו כמו רַדִין
'YRB' PWoLWNiYŠ [read: 'PWoLWNiYŠ]; it is a plant and its seeds are like RaDiYN

[20] אירבא פ״טיקולַארִיש ב״א ווילדא נעלכין
'YRB' FYṬYQWLa'RiYŠ; German WWYLD' N'LKYN

[21] אינקוֹבַ׳א שלְשִׁיקִיוֹם ב״א ווינגא וויזא והפרחי׳ שלה נקר׳ די אוניזייא
'YNQWoVa' [read: 'YNṬWoBa']; ŠLəŠiYQiYWoM; German WWYNG' [read: WWYG'] WWYZ'; its flowers are called DY 'WNYZYY'

[22] איפוקוויששטדוש ב״א שוומפא הגדל(?) במקו׳ הונדש רוזין
'YPWQWWYŠṬDWŠ; German ŠWWMP'; it grows at the [same] place [as] HWNDŠ RWZYN

בית
([Letter] Bet)[1]

[23] ברביוביש שטיקדוש ציטרינום הם פרחי׳ קטני׳ געלא ב״א וולא גמוט
BRBYWBYŠ; ŠṬYQDWŠ ṢYṬRYNWM; these are small G'L' (yellow) flowers; German WWL' GMWṬ

[24] ביריונייא ב״א ווילדא קורבש
BYRYWNYY'; German WWYLD' QWRBŠ

[25] ברקטיאוש שווינא ב״א זב״ין בום
BRQṬY'WŠ; ŠWWYN'; German ZVYN BWM

[26] בוגלושא ב״א אוהשן צונגא 12b
BWGLWŠ'; German 'WHŠN ṢWNG'

[27] בליטיש אורטוש ב״א אוהשין אווגין
BLYṬYŠ [read: BLYṬWŠ] 'WRṬWŠ; German 'WHŠYN 'WWGYN

[28] ברדנא לפא אינוֵורשַא מייאור ב״א גרושא לאטכא
BRDN'; LP' 'YNWWeRŠa'; MYY'WR; German GRWŠ' L'ṬK'

[29] בישטורטא אירבא בליטא ב״א מילדא
BYŠṬWRṬ'; 'YRB' BLYṬ'; German MYLD'

[30] בלֵיטַא ב״א מנגולט או רומשקולא
BLeYṬ'; German MNGWLṬ or RWMŠQWL'

[31] בורגו ב״א בורזא חם ולח במ״א
BWRGW; German BWRZ'; hot and moist in the first degree

1 The Ms has two mariginal entries: (1) ביצידין טִישְׁטִיקְלוּש—BYṢYDYN [read: BYṢY' HM(?)] ṬiYŠəṬiYQəLWŠ—BYṢY' (Hebrew) means 'testiculus' (Latin) (2) וולפש ב״א ראגארין—WWLPŠ; German R'G'RYN(?).

[32] ברונקוש קושקֻוטי עשב ב״א זידִי
BRWNQWŠ; QWŠQuWṬY; a plant [called] in German ZYDiY

[33] בזיליקא דרגנטיאה ב׳ שמו׳ לחד (*אחד) עשב
BZYLYQ'; DRGNṬY'H; two names for one and the same plant

[34] בישמלב׳א ב״א איביש
BYŠMLV'; German 'YBYŠ

אות גימל
(Letter Gimel)

[35] גניקוש ב״א זברון אין דעמא גרטין
GNYQWŠ; German ZBRWN 'YN D'M' GRṬYN

[36] גראמין ב״א וורצולא ב׳ון דעמא גרזין
GR'MYN; German WWRṢWL' [read: WWRṢL'] VWN D'M' GRZYN

[37] גלוקוש קושקוטא ב״א זידא
GLWQWŠ [read: GLWNQWŠ]; QWŠQWṬ'; German ZYD'

[38] גריאַה אוֹפִּלַטַא אוונציאה שַׁאנַא מוֹנְדַא ב״א בנדיקטא
GRY'aH 'WoPiLaṬa' [read: GRY'WoPiLaṬa']; 'WWNṢY'H; Ša'Na' MWoNəDa'; German BNDYQṬ'

אות דלת
(Letter Dalet)

[39] דורוניקא הוא שורש ויש קור׳ וורוניקא
DWRWNYQ'; i.e., a root; it is also called WWRWNYQ'

[40] דמניש ב״א לוראולי ב״ט אוליו לווארינום
DMNYŠ; German LWR'WLY; Latin 'WLYWo LWW'RYNWM

[41] דריגולס דרגנטיאה ב״א נטר וורצא
DRYGWLS [read: DRGNQWLS]; DRGNṬY'H; German NṬR WWRṢ'

[42] דינדו ליבנוס הפרח שלו נקר׳ אנטוש וי״א רוזמרינוס
DYNDW [read: DYNRDW] LYBNWS; the flower is called ’NṬWŠ; according to others RWZMRYNWS

[43] דיפראי פוליפודיון ב״א שטיין וור 13a
DYPR’Y [read: DYP’RY]; PWLYPWDYWN; German ŠṬYYN WWR [read: WWRṢ]

[44] דרדאנא ב״א רוש הופא
DRD’N’; German RWŠ HWP’

[45] דינְש אֵיקוונִיש שולפ׳ורטָא הוא עשב
DYNəŠ ’eYQWWNiYŠ [read: ’eYQWWNWŠ]; ŠWoLFWoRṬa’; i.e., a plant

[46] דקטלי הם גרעיני תמריי
DQṬLY; these are the kernels of dates

אות הא
(Letter He)

[47] היפא ב״א הונדש ביש
HYP’; German HWNDŠ BYŠ

אות ויו
(Letter Waw)

[48] ווירגא פשטוריש ב״א ווילדא קרטין
WWYRG’ PŠṬWRYŠ; German WWYLD’ QRṬYN

[49] וורוקרייא הוא עשב
WWRWQRYY’; i.e., a plant

[50] ורבינא ב״א איזר הרטא
WRBYN’; German ’YZR HRṬ’

אות זין
(Letter Zayin)

[51] זינזיבריש ב״א אינגבר
ZYNZYBRYŠ; German ʾYNGBR

[52] זיזנייא ראטא ב״א צוקר
ZYZNYYʾ; RʾṬʾ; German ṢWQR

[53] זיטוורייא הוא שורש
ZYṬWWRYYʾ; i.e., a root

אות טית
(Letter Ṭet)

[54] טמרישקוש י״א שהוא פרומא בוומא
ṬMRYŠQWŠ; some say that it is [German] PRWMʾ BWWMʾ

[55] טיטימלוש יש בו מיני׳ ו׳ ב״א וולפאש מילך
ṬYṬYMLWŠ; there are six varieties of it; German WWLPʾŠ MYLK

[56] טוטרביט הוא שורש
ṬWṬRBYṬ [read: ṬWRBYṬ]; i.e., a root

[57] טפשיאה הוא שורש שמנפחי׳ בו בני אדם
ṬPŠYʾH; i.e., a root that is used for swellings on people (?) (lit., that can cause swellings in people)

[58] טירוש הוא נחש
ṬYRWŠ; i.e., a snake

[59] טורמינטילא הוא עשב
ṬWRMYNṬYLʾ; i.e., a plant

[60] טרטרום ב״א ווין שטיין
ṬRṬRWM; German WWYN ŠṬYYN

אות יוד
(Letter Yod)

[61] יינשתולא יינישתי ב״א פרימן
YYNŠTWL'; YYNYŠTY; German PRYMN

אות למד
(Letter Lamed)

[62] לילי פאגוש ב״א ווילדא זלבא
LYLY P'GWŠ; German WWYLD' ZLB'

[63] ליפיטוש שפראטיש ב״א שטיין ברעכא זאמא
LiPYṬWŠ ŠPR'ṬYŠ [read: LiYṬW ŠPRM'ṬYŠ]; German ŠṬYYN BR'K' Z'M'

[64] ליבָא נוֹטִידש הוא עשב הנקר׳ רושמרינא 13b
LYBa' NWoṬiYDiŠ [read: NWoṬiYDoŠ]; i.e., a plant called RWŠMRYN'

[65] ליפוֹרִיש פְּרְאַפִּשְׁמוֹש שַׁטִירְיוֹן ה׳ עשב
LYPWoRiYŠ PəRi'aPiŠəMWoŠ [read: PəRi'aPiŠəQWoŠ]; ŠaṬiRəYWoN; i.e., a plant

[66] לוונדולא שלביא אגרישטיש ב״א ווילדא זלבא
LWWNDWL'; ŠLBY' 'GRYŠṬYŠ; German WWYLD' ZLB'

[67] לינוטִידִישְׁ מֵרְקוֹרְיָילֵיש ב״א שיש מילדא
LYNWṬiDiYŠə; MeRəQWoRəYYaLeYŠ; German ŠYŠ MYLD'

[68] לִינַרְיָא הוא עשב הדומה לאזולא מאד לא יתן חלב
LiYNaRəYa'; i.e., a plant that greatly resembles 'ZWL' [but] does not give milk

[69] ליליאום לגושטרום ב״א ווידא ווינדא
LYLY'WM; LGWŠṬRWM; German WWYD' WWYND'

[70] לינגום אביש ב״א ווגל צונגא
LYNGWM 'BYŠ; German WWGL ṢWNG'

[71] לאפציום אקוטי ב׳ מיני׳ גדול וקטן ב״א שפא שפיצין לאטנא(?)
L'PṢYWM 'QWṬY; two kinds: large and small; German ŠP' ŠPYṢYN L'ṬN'(?)

[72] לאפציום רטונדא ב״א רוש(?) הופא
L'PṢYWM RṬWND'; German RWŠ(?) HWP'

[73] ליטריירום ב״א האב׳ין ב׳ון זילְבֵר
LYṬRYYRWM; German H'VYN VWN ZYLəBeR

[74] לאַבְרון וונריש ב״א וויץ דישטל
L'aBəRWN [read: L'aBəRWM] WWNRYŠ; German WWYṢ DYŠṬL

[75] למנייאש ב״א אורפימנטום
LMNYY'Š; German 'WRPYMNṬWM

[76] לקא ב״א גומא שצובעי׳ בו אדום
LQ'; German GWM'; that is used as a red dye

[77] לקטירידיש קאטפוציא שם עשב ושם זרע ב״א שפרינקא וורצא
LQṬYRYDYŠ; Q'ṬPWṢY'; the name of a plant and the name of a seed; German ŠPRYNQ' WWRṢ'

[78] לופולוס ב״א הופא
LWPWLWS; German HWP'

[79] לאוריַאלא ציגלינדא ב״א צידלבשט
L'WRYa'L'; [German] ṢYGLYND'; German ṢYDLBŠṬ

[80] לינליאוֹן ב״א לין אוליי
LYNLY'WoN; German LYN 'WLYY

14a **[אות מים]**
[Letter Mem]

[81] מירטוש והזרע שלו מֶרְטֵליש והשמן נקר׳ ב״ט אוליו מֶרְטֵלי
MYRṬWŠ; its seed is MeRəṬeLYŠ; and its oil is called in Latin 'WLYW [read: 'WLYWM] MeRəṬeLY

[82] מרוֹביוֹם פְּרַצְיוֹם ב״א אנדורן
MRWoBYWoM; PəRaṢəYWoM; German ’NDWRN

[83] מציש ב״א מושקדון בלומין
MṢYŠ; German MWŠQDWN BLWMYN

[84] מאבַ׳אמַטיקום ב״א קול שתחתיו לבן
M’Va’MaṬYQWM [read: M’Va’BeMaṬYQWM]; German QWL that is white at the base

[85] מילפולייא אמברוזייא מינא ב״א גרווא
MYLPWLYY’ [read: MYLPWLY’WM] ’MBRWZYY’ MYN’; German GRWW’

[86] מרְשִׁילְיוֹם פַּאבַ׳א לופֵּינַא ב״א נהט שדא
MRəŠiYLəYWoM; Pa’Va’ LWPeYNa’; German NHṬ ŠD’

[87] מיקוֹניוֹם אוֹק קוֹמִדַא ב״א וויש מגזאמא
MYQWoNYWoM ’WoQ QWoMiDa’; German WWYŠ MGZ’M’

[88] מנגניש ב״א אבן המושך ברזל
MNGNYŠ in German; a stone that attracts iron

[89] מאלַא שִׁילוֶוֶשְׁטִרִייַא ב״א אֵפל צמא אונ׳ ווילדא הנקר׳ הולצאֵפל
M’La’ ŠiYLWWeŠəṬiRiYYa’; German ’ePL ṢM’ ’WN’ WWYLD’, which are called HWLṢ’ePL

[90] מריקא ייֵנִישתַא ב״א חיילא אונ׳ פראמא
MRYQ’; YYeNiYŠTa’; German ḤYYL’ [read: ḤYYD’] and PR’M’

[91] מיאטיש הוא עשב זר
MY’ṬYŠ; i.e., a foreign plant

[92] מישְׁפִּלַא ב״א מישפולן
MYŠPiLa’; German MYŠPWLN

[93] מושקוש ב״א ביזימא
MWŠQWŠ; German BYZYM’ [read: BYZM’]

[94] מוזַא הוא פרי אילן הנמצא בירושלי׳
MWZa'; i.e., the fruit of a tree that [grows] in Jerusalem

[95] מציום ב״א מִנְיוּם
MṢYWM [read: MṢYNWM]; German MiNəYWM

[96] מושִׁילֵיאוֹן הוא שמן עשוי מן ביזמא
MWŠiYLeY'WoN [read: MWŠṢeYLeY'WoN]; i.e., oil produced from BYZM'

[97] מילפודיום ב״א בלי
MYLPWDYWM [read: MWLYPDYNWM]; German BLY

[98] מירִיאוֹן אורקְלַאמוֹרִיש ב״א מוז אורא
MYRiY'WoN; 'WRQəLa'MWoRiYŠ; German MWZ 'WR'

14b **אות נון**
(Letter Nun)

[99] נינפֵיאה הוא עשב הגדל במים
NYNPeY'H; i.e., a plant that grows in the water

[100] נרקוש הוא דג וִוִשְׁא אונ׳ זין שלם(?) מכט שלפן
NRQWŠ; i.e., a WWiŠə' (white) fish; 'WN' ZYN ŠLM(?) MKṬ ŠLPN

[101] נַאפָּא פִּטִרוליוֹן הוא מין שמן אונ׳ אישט רוטא ב׳רווא
Na'Pa' [read: Na'PṬa']; PiṬiRWLYWoN; i.e., a kind of oil; 'WN' 'YŠṬ RWṬ' [read: RWṬ'R] VRWW'

[102] נוקליאוש הם פיניין קורנר
NWQLY'WŠ; i.e., PYNYYN QWRNR

[103] ניניאוש ב״א זֵמְדְא ורמיילגלגן(?)
NYNY'WŠ [read: NYLY'WŠ(?)]; German ZeMəDə'; WRMYYLGLGN(?)

אות סמך
(Letter Samekh)

[104] סאגפינום שיראפינום ⟨והוא גומא⟩
S'GPYNWM ŠYR'PYNWM; [i.e., gum]

[105] סזיליום שילריש מונטעניש הוא זרע
SZYLYWM; ŠYLRYŠ MWNṬ'NYŠ; i.e., a seed

[106] שקווינגטום הוא מין שטרוֹ
ŠQWWYNNṬWM; i.e., a kind of ŠṬRWo

[107] סטיקדוש ב׳ מיני׳ והם געלין בלומין ב״א וולגמוט
SṬYQDWŠ; two kinds; i.e., G'LYN BLWMYN; German WWLGMWṬ

[108] סטיריון הוא עשב
SṬYRYWN; i.e., a plant

[109] סאביוזא הוא עשב
S'BYWZ' [read: SQ'BYWZ']; i.e., a plant

[110] סניקון קרדו בנדיקטוש ב״א קרוצוורץ
SNYQWN [read: SNYQYWN]; QRDW [read: QRDWŠ] BNDYQṬWŠ; German QRWṢWWRṢ

[111] סינַאצוֹ ב״א ב⟨רונען⟩ קרעשא
SYNa'ṢWo [read: SYNa'ṢYWo]; German B[RWN'N] QR'Š'

[112] סנדלי הם ג׳ מינים רוט וויש געלא
SNDLY; there are three varieties of them: RWṬ (red), WWYŠ (white), G'L' (yellow)

[113] סרְפֵלוֹם חַרְפִילוֹם הוא עשב פליחשט(?) אין דער ער⟨.⟩ן
SRəPeLWoM; ḤaRəPiYLWoM [read: HaRəPiLWoM]; i.e., a plant PLYḤŠṬ(?) 'YN D'R 'R[.]N

[114] סנטווריאה הוא עשב
SNṬWWRY'H; i.e., a plant

[115] ספִּירְמַא הוא זרע
SPeYRəMa'; i.e., a seed (sperm)

15a [116] סטונבילי ב״א פניין קורנר
SṬWNBYLY [read: SṬRWBYLY]; German PNYYN QWRNR

[117] סיקומורוש פיקוש פאטואה הוא אילן והפרי שלו נקר׳ ציקא מינא
SYQWMWRWŠ; PYQWŠ P'ṬW'H; i.e., a tree, and its fruit is called ṢYQ' MYN'

[118] סקורפייא הוא חיה קטנ׳ ויש לו ארס
SQWRPYY'; it is a small poisonous animal

[119] סיליום שוטה מעריי הוא עשב
SYLYWM ŠWṬH [read: SYGYLWM ŠNṬH] M'RYY; i.e., a plant

[120] שמיריוש ביטוניקא ב״א בטונייא
ŠMYRYWŠ [read: ŠMYRNYŠ]; BYṬWNYQ'; German BṬWNYY'

[121] סישטור הוא אניטום אגרישטי ב״א ווילדא טיל
SYŠṬWR; i.e., 'NYṬWM 'GRYŠṬY; German WWYLD' ṬYL

[122] סלינום ב״א אֶפא זאמא
SLYNWM; German 'eP' Z'M'

[123] סִיכֶן ב״א ווילדא עברצין
SiYKeN; German WWYLD' 'BRṢYN

[124] סקריאולא אנדיב׳ייא ב״א זו דישטל
SQRY'WL'; 'NDYVYY'; German ZW DYŠṬL

[125] סאפונרייא הוא עשב ויש לו זרע כמו רַדִין
S'PWNRYY'; i.e., a plant that has a seed like RaDiYN

[126] סולפ׳וראטא הוא עלה של מים
SWLFWR'Ṭ'; i.e., a water [plant](?) (lit., "leaf")

אות פה
(Letter Pe)

[127] פילי פנדולא יש לו בשורש כמו ב׳ בצים
PYLY PNDWL'; in its roots it has something similar to two testicles

[128] פינצייא ב״א דייטלא
PYNṢYY'; German DYYṬL'

[129] פִלוֹשְׁא צִירִיאַקוֹש ב״א באפל
PiLWoŠə' ṢiYRiY'aQWoŠ [read: ṢiYRiY'aQWuŠ]; German B'PL

[130] פניקולטא הוא עשב ארוך וגדל במים
PNYQWLṬ'; it is a large plant that grows in the water

[131] פניגריקא ונקר׳ כן ב״א
PNYGRYQ'; it is called similarly in German

[132] פלושְׁמֵ⟨...⟩ ווילדא ויש לו פרחים׳ געלא
PLWŠəMe[...]; WWYLD'; and it has flowers [that are] G'L' (yellow)

[133] פוליום ב״א בְלֵדֵר מנעלכין
PWLYWM; German BəLeDeR MN'LKYN

[134] פלַאוירא הוא עשב מר וטוב בפני התולעי׳
PLa'WYR' [read: PLa'WR']; i.e., a plant that is bitter and good against worms

[135] פאב׳א הוא עשב
P'V'; i.e., a plant

[136] פלִקְטִינא בוֹלְבַא הוא עשב 15b
PLiQəṬiYN'; BWoLəBa'; i.e., a plant

[137] פלְטַרֵי ב״א טוזינט גילדין
PLəṬaReY [read: PLəṬeReY]; German ṬWZYNṬ GYLDYN

[138] פלִיקִיש קוורצינאה הוא פוליפודיוֹ
PLiYQiYŠ QWWRṢYN'H; i.e., PWLYPWDYWo

[139] פירוֹגוֹ פֵּירַרְיוּם ב״א דש מאן בינדיט אימליש טרוג
PYRWoGWo; PeYRaRəYWM; German DŠ M'N BYNDYṬ 'YMLYŠ ṬRWG

[140] פאויצִידְנוּש וֵנִיקלוּש פורצינוש הוא עשב
P'WYṢiYDəNWŠ [read: P'WYṢeDaNWŠ]; WWeNiYQLWŠ PWRṢYNWŠ; i.e., a plant

[141] פאלִיקַרְיַיא ב״א נהט אונ׳ טאק
P'LiYQaRəYYa' [read: P'LiYṬaRiYYa']; German NHṬ 'WN' Ṭ'Q

[142] פשִׁילִיוֹם הוא עשב ונקר׳ גם פוֹלִיטַרְיַא ויש קורי׳ אותו פַּלְמַא קְרִישְׁטֵי וכשמושחים בו הידים עם המיץ ישאו ברזל חם בלתי כויה
PŠiYLYWoM; i.e., a plant that is also called PWoLiYṬaRəYa' [read: PWaLiYQaRəYa'] and also PaLəMa' QəRiYŠəṬeY [read: QəRiYŠəṬiY]; if one rubs its juice on one's hands one can lift hot iron without getting burned

[143] פרִיאַפִּיש ב״א מנשא דצקא
PRiY'aPiYŠ [read: PRiY'aPWuŠ]; German MNŠ' DṢQ' [read: ṢQL]

[144] פינטוֹדַקְטְלִיש קושטוש הוא עשב
PYNṬWoDaQəṬəLiYŠ; QWŠṬWŠ; i.e., a plant

[145] פַּאכִּיטַרְיַיא פַּרִיצִיַיאדוש עשב
Pa'KiYṬaRəYYa' [read: Pa'RiYṬaRəYYa']; PaRiYṢiYYa'DWŠ [read: PaRiYṢiYDiYa'DWŠ]; a plant

[146] פאליוֹם רֵיגַלֵי אֵלִיקוּנִיוֹם ב״א פוליי ויש מין נקר׳ פוליי צִרְוִוינוּם
P'LYWoM ReYGaLeY; 'eLiYQWNiYWoM [read: GLiYQWNiYWoM]; German PWLYY; there is a variety that is called PWLYY ṢiRWWiYNWM [read: ṢeRWWiYNWM]

[147] פרַשִׁיוֹם מַרוֹבְיוֹם אלבום ב״א אנדורן
PRaŠiYWoM; MaRWoBəYWoM 'LBWM; German 'NDWRN

[148] פניקוֹלש שְׁפוֹן ייאַה ב״א מֵרְשווַמפא
PNYQWoLŠ; ŠəPWoN YY'aH; German MeRəŠWWaMP'

[149] פליגונייא פוֹלִיגְנְיוֹם ב״א וועגא טרעטא
PLYGWNYY'; PWoLiYGəNəYWoM; German WW'G' ṬR'Ṭ'

[150] פִּירִישְׁטִרוּרִי אוֹרטוֹן בִּירבֵּינַא רִיקְטַא ב״א איזר הרטא
PYRiYŠṬiRWRY [read: PYRiYŠṬeReWoN] ʾWoRṬWoN; ViRBeYNaʾ RiYQəṬaʾ [read: ReYQəṬa]; German ʾYZR HRṬʾ

[151] פִּינְטַאפִּילוֹן ב״א ב׳ונף ב׳ינגר
PiYNəṬaʾPiYLWN; German VWNP VYNGR

[152] פְּרַאפּוֹלִיוֹן ב״א וויש ווהשא 16a
PRaPWoLiYWoN [read: PRoPWoLiYWoN]; German WWYŠ WWHŠʾ

[153] פיפנעלְא ב״א ביבינעלא ודומ׳ לשַׁקְשִׁיפְּרְגא
PYPNʿLəʾ [read: PYPYNʿLʾ]; German BYBYNʿLʾ; it is similar to ŠaQəŠiYPəRəGʾ

[154] פלאטא ב״א שילריש מונטעניש
PLʾṬʾ; German ŠYLRYŠ MWNṬʿNYŠ

[155] פיקוש ב״א וויש בעכא
PYQWŠ; German WWYŠ BʿKʾ

[156] פשידייא ב״א שֵׁלוֹטְא ב׳ון גרנט אֶפל
PŠYDYYʾ; German ŠeLWoṬəʾ VWN GRNṬ ʾePL

[157] פיפְּלוֹם ב״א שטינבדא דישטל
PYPəLWoM; German ŠṬYNBDʾ DYŠṬL

[158] פלִינִיוֹם הוא עשב
PLYNYWoM [read: PLYṢiYNWoM]; i.e., a plant

[159] פְּרֵיצִיאַדוֹש הוא שיש מעלדא
PReYṢiYʾaDWoŠ [read: PeRDYṢiʾaDWoŠ]; i.e., ŠYŠ MʿLDʾ

אות צדי
(Letter Ṣade)

[160] צִינאגלוֹשא ב״א הונש צונגא
ṢYNʾGLWoŠʾ; German HWNŠ ṢWNGʾ

[161] צִילִידוֹנְיַיא אגרישטיש ב״א ווילדא שֶׁלְווְרצא
ṢYLiYDWoNəYYa’ ’GRYŠṬYŠ; German WWYLD’ ŠeLəWWRəṢ’

[162] צימְבַלַרְיַא אוֹמליקש הוא עשב גדל בקירות
ṢYMBaLaRəYa’ [read: ṢYMBaLaRiYa’]; ’WoMLYQŠ; i.e., a plant that grows on walls

[163] צִיקלַאמִין ב״א ערדא נושא
ṢYQLa’MiYN; German ‘RD’ NWŠ’

אות קוף
(Letter Qof)

[164] קונדִיקוֹש ב״א שִׁלוֹטְא ב׳ון ווישר ניזא ווירצא
QWNDiYQWoŠ [read: QWNDYiŠYi]; German ŠiLWoṬə’ VWN WWYŠR NYZ’ WWYRṢ’

[165] קוזון ב״א עביך קוזון אֶדְרַא
QWZWN [read: QYZWN]; German ‘BYK; QWZWN [read: QYZWN]; ’eDəRa’

[166] קוֹקוֹנדְיוֹן הוא זרע מן צידלבשט
QWoQWoNDəYWoN [read: QWoQWoNiDiYWoN]; i.e., seed from [German] ṢYDLBŠṬ

[167] קאניקוֹלַטַא קאני קוֹלַרִיש יושקווימי ב״א בולזין זאמין
Q’NYQWoLaṬa’; Q’NY QWoLaRYŠ; YWŠQWWYMY; German BWLZYN [read: BYLZYN] Z’MYN

[168] קלמוש ארומטיקוש הוא שורש עשב
QLMWŠ ’RWMṬYQWŠ; i.e., the root of a plant

[169] קרשולא ב״א שטיין פעפר
QRŠWL’; German ŠṬYYN P‘PR

[170] קרפו בלשמ׳ הוא פרי מן האילן
QRPW BLŠM’; i.e., the fruit of the tree

[171] קְרְדוּמֵנִי קרווי אגרישטי ב״א מט קומל 17a[2]
QRəDWMeNY; QRWWY ’GRYŠṬY; German MṬ QWML

[172] קרוֹנוּפוֹדְיוֹן פֵּיש צֶרְבִ׳ינוֹס הוא עשב ב״א היריש ווש
QRWoNWoPWoDəYWoN; PeYŠ ṢeRəViYNWoS; i.e., a plant; German HYRYŠ [read: HYRŠ] WWŠ [read: VWŠ]

[173] קְרִיזוֹלִימָא בלשוֹ׳ פרוב׳נצא אתרוג
QRiYZWoLiYMa’; in the language of PRWVNṢ’ (Provence(?)) ’TRWG (i.e., Hebrew for citron)

[174] קְרִיַּאַקָא פַּשְׁטִינַקָא ב״א ווילדא מורהין
QRiYYa’aQa’ [read: QRiYYoQa’]; PaŠəṬiYNaQa’; German WWYLD’ MWRHYN

[175] קַרַמְבִיַּא ב״א איי⟨...⟩הַנְדא וויש קול
QRaMəBYYa’; German ’YY[...]HaNəD’ WWYŠ QWL

[176] קְלְמִינטא ב״א שטיין מינצא
QLəMiYNṬ’; German ŠṬYYN MYNṢ’

[177] קְמִילִיאוֹנְטַא הוא עשב שמעמידי׳ בו חלב
QMiYLiY’WoNəṬ’; i.e., a plant from which [curdled] milk is obtained

[178] קרישפּוּלא א׳ ב(?) צֶנְטוֹם גַרְנא ב״א הונדרט קורנר
QRYŠPWuL’ ’’ B(?) ṢeNəṬWoM GRaN’; German HWNDRṬ QWRNR

[179] קרוקוש אוֹרְיֵינִטַליש ב״א זפרון
QRWQWŠ ’WoRəYYeNiṬaLYŠ; German ZPRWN

[180] קרוקוש אוֹרְטֵנְצִיש ב״א ווילדא זפרון
QRWQWŠ ’WoRəṬeNəṢiYŠ; German WWYLD’ ZPRWN

[181] קוניאום צִיקוטא ב״א עשב שערלינקא
QWNY’WM; ṢiYQWṬ’; in German the plant [called] Š‘RLYNQ’

2 Fol. 16b is not part of the glossary. It begins with a lengthy recipe, the first part of which is missing, and then gives a variety of short recipes for a.o. ארפע (herpes), bad breath, and removing freckles.

[182] קרְפוֹפְשִׁי פרוקטוש אֶדְרֵי הם פרי הגדל על עבך
QRəPWoPiŠiY [read: QRəPWoṢiŠiY]; PRWQṬWŠ ʾeDəReY; i.e., fruit that grows on ʿBK

[183] קרוֹאֵי אגְרִישְׁטֵי ב״א ווילדא מט קומל
QRWoʾeY ʾGəRiYŠəṬeY; German WWYLDʾ MṬ QWML

[184] קושטוש אורטרוֹם ב״א גְראש לַטְכְא
QWŠṬWŠ ʾWRṬRWoM; German GəRʾŠ LaṬəKəʾ

[185] קולוקווִינְטְדֵי הוא קוֹקוֹרביטא אלכסנדרינא
QWLWQWWiYNəṬəDeY; i.e., QWoQWoRBYṬʾ ʾLKSNDRYNʾ

[186] קוֹדִיוֹם הוא ב״א שוורצא מגאולִיי
QWoDiYWoM; i.e., German ŠWWRṢʾ MGʾWLiYY

אות ריש
(Letter Resh)

[187] רודון ב״א רוזא
RWDWN; German RWZʾ

[188] רוֹדוֹשְׁטוֹמַא ב״א רוזן וושר אוקשי רודון הוא אֵשיק און׳ רוזין אוליי גמישט
RWoDWoŠəṬoMaʾ; German RWZN WWŠR; ʾWQŠY RWDWN; i.e., ʾeŠYQ ʾWNʾ RWZYN ʾWLYY GMYŠṬ

[189] רוי הוא ריברבא
RWY; i.e., RYBRBʾ [read: RYWBRBʾR]

[190] רוֹש צִרְיַיקוֹש ב״א בפלא בלומין
RWoŠ ṢiRəYYaQWoŠ; German BPLʾ BLWMYN

[191] רישטא בוב׳יש
RYŠṬʾ BWVYŠ

17b [192] רוֹמֶקְש הוא ב׳ מיני׳ אחד יש לו פרי והשני לא
RWoMeQəŠ; it consists of two kinds, one has fruits and the other not

[193] רזִינַא כל גומא נקר׳ כן וכשכותבי׳ כך בלא דבר אז הוא אותו גומ׳ הבא מן הַטנְא חזק
RZiYN'; every gum is called by that name; when it is written without any [specification] it means that gum that comes from the ṬNə'

Be strong [and resolute; do not be terrified and dismayed, for the Lord your God is with you wherever you go].[3]

3 Cf. Joshua 1:9. Translation JPS.

Reconstruction of Latin and German Terms

Abbreviations

Alphita = García González, Alejandro (ed.), *Alphita: Edición crítica y comentario*, Florence 2007 (Edizione Nazionale “La Scuola Medica Salernitana,” vol. 2) (references to an entry consist of letter + number, others are to pages; in rare cases, we cite Mss of *Alphita* with their sigla in italics as reported by García González).

André = André, Jacques, *Les noms de plantes dans la Rome antique*, Paris 1985 (Collection d'études anciennes).

CGL = *Corpus glossariorum Latinorum*, ed. by G. Goetz, vols. 1–5, Lipsiae 1888–1923.

Daems = Daems, Willem F., *Nomina simplicium medicinarum ex synonymariis medii aevi collecta: Semantische Untersuchungen zum Fachwortschatz hoch- und spätmittelalterlicher Drogenkunde*, Leiden-New York-Köln 1993 (Studies in Ancient Medicine, vol. 6) (references are to numbered entries [lemmata], where Daems usually gives [without further discussion] a modern equivalent in botanical nomenclature and German).

DMLBS = *Dictionary of Medieval Latin from British Sources*, online at https://logeion.uchicago.edu.

Fischer = Fischer, Hermann, *Mittelalterliche Pflanzenkunde*, Repr., Hildesheim 1967 (reference is made to pages).

García González, see Alphita.

Goltz = Goltz, Dietlinde, *Studien zur Geschichte der Mineralnamen in Pharmazie, Chemie und Medizin von den Anfängen bis Paracelsus*, Wiesbaden 1972 (Sudhoffs Archiv, suppl. 14).

Grimm = Grimm, Jacob und Wilhelm, *Deutsches Wörterbuch*, 1854–1971, digitale Ausgabe des Kompetenzzentrums für elektronische Erschließungs- und Publikationsverfahren in den Geisteswissenschaften der Universität Trier (online at woerterbuchnetz.de/DWB/).

Haars = Haars, Maximilian, *Die allgemeinen Wirkungspotenziale der einfachen Arzneimittel bei Galen: Oreibasios, Collectiones medicae XV*, Stuttgart 2018 (Quellen und Studien zur Geschichte der Pharmazie, vol. 116).

Hildegard, Physica = Hildegard von Bingen, *Physica*, Edition der Florentiner Handschrift (Cod. Laur. Ashb. 1323, ca. 1300) … von Irmgard Müller und Christian Schulze unter Mitarbeit von Sven Neumann, Hildesheim 2008.

Lexer = Matthias Lexer, *Mittelhochdeutsches Handwörterbuch*, 3 vols., Leipzig 1872–1878 (online at woerterbuchnetz.de/Lexer).

Marzell = Marzell, Heinrich, *Wörterbuch der deutschen Pflanzennamen*, 5 vols., Leipzig 1937–1958.

 | DOI:10.1163/9789004459380_005

Mensching = Mensching, Guido, *La sinonima delos nonbres delas medeçinas griegos e latynos e arauigos*, estudio y edición crítica, Madrid 1994.

MHG = Middle High German

MLW = *Mittellateinisches Wörterbuch bis zum ausgehenden 13. Jahrhundert*, München 1967 ff. (A–C = vols. 1–2, online at woerterbuchnetz.de/MLW/[1]; the PDF of D–H = vols. 3–4, is available at http://www.mlw.badw.de/mlw-digital/mlw-open-access.html).

Rufinus = *The Herbal of Rufinus*, ed. from the unique manuscript by L. Thorndike, ass. by F.S. Benjamin Jr., Chicago 1949.

Stirling = Stirling, János, *Lexicon nominum herbarum, arborum fruticumque linguae Latinae, ex fontibus Latinitatis ante saeculum XVII scriptis collegit et descriptionibus botanicis illustravit Iohannes Stirling*, I–IV, ex aedibus domus editoriae Encyclopaedia Budapestini 1995–1998.

ThlL = *Thesaurus linguae Latinae*, http://publikationen.badw.de/de/thesaurus/lemmata.

Ventura = *Ps. Bartholomaeus Mini de Senis, Tractatus de herbis* (Ms London, British Library, Egerton 747), a cura di Iolanda Ventura, Florence 2009 (Edizione Nazionale "La Scuola Medica Salernitana," vol. 5) (quoted with the number of the entry and, if necessary, the note of the commentary).

Winkler = Winkler, Joachim, *Physicae quae fertur Plinii Florentino-Pragensis liber primus*, Frankfurt a. M.-Bern 1984 (Lateinische Sprache und Literatur des Mittelalters, vol. 17).

1 At the same URL woerterbuchnetz.de, a number of German dictionaries can be searched at the same time, e.g., Lexer's *Mittelhochdeutsches Handwörterbuch* (Lexer), and *Frühneuhochdeutsches Wörterbuch* (FWB), which are relevant for our purposes, as well as MHG dictionaries or dictionaries of German dialects, e.g., *Südhessisches Wörterbuch* (SHW).

Glossary 1

	Latin	German	Grimm	Notes
1	eupatorium (epatorium)	wilde silbe	wildsalbei	Ventura 162 calidum est in primo gradu, siccum in secundo, cf. below 110. MLW s.v. eupatorium 2a, Stirling s.v. eupatoria 4.
2	emblici (emblici)	winstain	weinstein	Ventura 163 enblici fructus sunt ⟨in⟩ ultramarinis partibus crescentis. *emblici* (cf. DMLBS), however, cannot mean weinstein.
3	endiuia (endiuie)	wize distel	*weiszdistel	Ventura 158 frigida est et sicca in primo gradu.
4	enula (emila[2])	alant	alant	Ventura 160 calida est in fine tertii gradus, humida in principio. Grimm alant (2). Cf. below 11 and 98.
5a	epithymum (ipitimi)			Ventura 159 epithimum calidum est et siccum in tertio gradu.
5b	thymum (timi)			
6	euphorbium (eforbiun)			Ventura 161 calidum est et siccum in quarto gradu. Cf. 29.
7	epatica (epatice)	leber krut	leberkraut	Ventura 164 frigida est et sicca in primo gradu.
8	es ustum (es ustum)	glizistain	glitzigstein	Ventura 165 calidum est et siccum in quarto gradu. Cf. Grimm s.v. glasstein; glitzerstein is not identified with anything real.
9	helleborus (eliborum)	nise wirze	nieswurz	Ventura 167. Cf. 46 below.
10	esula minor, esula maior (esula minora,[3] maior)			Ventura 168. Only the first two species can be identified; the text names just four and not, as announced, five species. Stirling

2 Cf. Stirling s.v. inula 1, DMLBS s.v. inula c, Daems 190 (where the forms emilla and immilla seem acceptable), Mensching 76,44.

3 The -a in minora is probably an error of transmission.

(*cont.*)

	Latin	German	Grimm	Notes
				and Daems 196/571 are of no help for the identification of the last two. Cf. 99 below.
11	enula (e⟨n⟩ula)			Already in 4 above.
12	eruca (eruca)			Cf. Daems 419, Stirling s.v. eruca; Grimm s.v. senf 5); Ventura 169 n. 1 wiz senff; cf. 74 below.
12a	erucula (erucol)			
13	ebulus (ebulus)	atik	attich	Ventura 171 calidus est et siccus. Cf. 97 below.
14	gentiana (enciane[4])	enzeon	enzian	Ventura 201 calida est et sicca in tertio gradu. Cf. 164 below.
15	hermodactylus (ermodactilus)	helehobit	helhop	Ventura 223 calidi sunt et sicci in tertio gradu. Hildegard, Physica; Marzell helhop; heilhobit; Fischer 265; cf. 50 below.
16	[ispe]	ysope	ysop	ispe is German, cf. Grimm s.v. ysop. Ventura 232 calidus est et siccus in tertio gradu.
17	iris (ireos)	blalilien	blaulilie	blâ is the older form of 'blau'; cf. 51, 62 and 95 below. Ventura 234 calidus est et siccus in secundo gradu.
18	iuniperus (iniperum)	⟨wachol⟩-derbeeren	wacholder-beere	Daems 262. Ventura 236 calidus est et siccus in tertio gradu.
19	ocimum (ozimum[5])	basilien-same	basiliensame	O1. Daems 350. Ventura 339 calidum est et siccum. Cf. 54 below.
20	opium (opium)			Ventura 341 frigidum est in quarto gradu, siccum in primo. Dried opium juice could be said to resemble a gum.
20a	gumma (guma)			

4 This may be a German, not a Latin form; it is neither attested in MLW nor in DMLBS.

5 This confirms the spelling ozimum; cf. DMLBS s.v. ocimum.

(*cont.*)

	Latin	German	Grimm	Notes
21	origanum (origanum)	doste	dost	Ventura 342 calidum est et siccum in tertio gradu.
22	oxylapathum (oxilapaci[a])	sura anfer	sauerampfer	
23	hordeum (orteum)	gerstenmel	gerstenmehl	Ventura 345 frigidum est et siccum.
24	os de corde cerui (osis de corde [a]cerui)	benken	beinchen	Ventura 346. bein 'bone'; 'from the heart of a deer' is omitted in the German.
25	os sepie (osis sepie)			Ventura 349 frigide et sicce complexionis est.
26	olibanum (olibanum)	wirok	weihrauch	Ventura 350 calidum est et siccum in secundo gradu.
27	apium (apii)	eppe	eppich	Ventura 8 calidum est in principio tertii gradi [sic!], siccum in medio eiusdem.
28	asarum (asari)	haselwirze	haselwurz	Ventura 46 calida est et sicca in tertio gradu.
29	euphorbium (eforbi)			Ventura 161 calidum est et siccum in quarto gradu. Cf. 6.
30	anethum (aneti)	tille	dill (tyl)	Ventura 16 calidum est et siccum in secundo gradu.
31	anisum (anisi)	anis	anis	Ventura 21 calidum est et siccum in tertio gradu.
32	alipta muscata (alipte muscade)			A123 Alipta quedam confectio est ... que dicitur alipta muscata. Mensching 67,2.
33	opopanax (apopanac)			F16 (app. crit.) opopanac; apo- also attested, cf. MLW and Mensching 110,26.
34	absinthium (apsintiun)	wermute	wermut	Cf. 47.
34a	apsincium (apsinciun)			

(*cont.*)

	Latin	German	Grimm	Notes
35	*uncertain*			Since it is called a gum, the first syllable may be opo-. With Mensching p. 134 n. 8 "opocici (?) M", perhaps opocicum (or rather apo-), and cf. Daems 200 apocissi edere gummi.
36	anacardium (anacardi)	helfantlus	elefantenlaus	A73 anacardus pediculus elefantis. Ventura 23 calidi sunt et sicci in tertio gradu.
37	*uncertain*	*uncertain*		
38	acorus (acori)	gele lilien	gelbe lilie	Grimm s.v. gelb 2b).
39	aristologia (aristolongie)	oster luzien	osterluzei	Ventura 27.
40	ameos (amei[6])			Ventura 52 uirtutem habet calidam et siccam in tertio gradu.
41	amomum (amomi[7])	wilde peter?	wilde petersilie	The German is uncertain. Ventura 53 calidum est et siccum in tertio gradu.
42	*uncertain*			KSP ḤY is not German but Hebrew for 'mercury'.
43	albe margarite (albarum margaritarum)	dingelkrut?		Cf. Ventura 298; dingelkraut (usually: dingel) cannot be a translation of 'white pearls'.
44	herba perforata (erbe porforate)	iohanis krut	johanniskraut	Cf. 48 below.
45	schoenanthus (esquinanti[8])	kemelenkrut howe	kamelkraut, kamelheu	Daems 445. Ventura 426 calidum est et siccum in tertio gradu. Cf. Grimm. s.v. kamelheu and below 276.

6 The gen. of Greek ἄμ(μ)ι is ἄμεως, transliterated as *ameos* and *ameus*, from which later a (spurious) Latin genitive *amei* is formed.

7 Daems 365 sinomum, wild petterly, if amomi is an error for sinoni, cf. Mensching 147,14 and n. 65.

8 The form with e- would belong to the Romance area. See below on 65.

(*cont.*)

	Latin	German	Grimm	Notes
46	helleborus (elibo-rum)	nise wurz	nieswurz	Cf. 9 above. Ventura 167 calidus est et siccus in tertio gradu.
47	absinthium (apsen-ciu⟨n⟩)	wermut	wermut	Ventura 22 calidum est et siccum in secundo gradu. Cf. 34.
47a	absincium (asin-ciu⟨n⟩)			For as- cf. MLW 1. absinthium.
48	hypericum (iperi-cun)	iohanis krut	johan-niskraut	Cf. 44 above.
49	abrotanum (abrotanum)	stabe wurz	stabwurz	
50	hermodactylus (ermodactilum)	hail hobet	helhop	Cf. 15 above. (The reading hail hobte seems less likely.)
51	iris (iris)	lilien wiz		Grimm only has weiszlilie; cf. 17 and 62 below.
52	hepatica (epaticum)	leber krut	leberkraut	Stirling also lists hepaticum.
53	artemisia (artemisia)	bibos	beifusz	Daems 1. Ventura 30 uirtutem habet calidam et siccam in tertio gradu.
54	ocimum (ozimum)	frisilain	*frieslein	Cf. 19 above and plant names con-taining fries- in Marzell.
55	ammoniacum (armoniacum)			Here, rock salt (sal gemme), not the gum, cf. MLW s.v. Ammoniacus.
56	antimonium (*anti-mosa)	bli esche	bleiasche	Different meaning in Grimm. Ven-tura 13 calidum est et siccum in quarto gradu. Cf. 89.
57	*uncertain*	… salz		
58	hypocistis (ipoqui-stidos)	hundis rose	hundsrose	I6. Daems 404. The German word refers to the fungus that grows on the rosa canina.
59	herba *uncertain* (irbe blaci)	milte muter	*milde mut-ter?	
60	amylum (amidum)			Ventura 12 temperate calidum et humidum.
61	orobus (orobi)	wikin	wicke	Ventura 524 calidum est in primo gradu, siccum in secundo.

(*cont.*)

	Latin	German	Grimm	Notes
62	iris (ireos)	wislilien	weiszlilie	Also called 'white' in 51 above, whereas in 17 and 95 it is called 'blue'; the colour of the flowers varies.
63	asparagus[9] (isparagi)			Identification not certain; while known in antiquity, our asparagus was perhaps not used in Germany during the middle ages.
63a	bruscus (brusci)			Asparagus officinalis does have male and female plants; the identification of bruscus and asparagus (as in a gloss, Ventura 84 n. 3) is doubtful.
64	urtica[10] (urtice)	nesele	nessel	
65	spodium (espodium[11])	gebrant helfen zene	gebranntes elfenbein	MHG helfenbein; Ventura 434 n. 1; Goltz, p. 133. Daems 444.
66	squilla (esquele)	mer zwibel	meerzwiebel	Ventura 454 calida est et sicca in secundo gradu. Cf. 266 below.
67		iwisch	eibisch	Ventura 292 calidus est et humidus in secundo gradu.
68	ebulus (ebuli)	*arebe?		Ventura 171 calidus est et siccus.
69	asa fetida (asafetide[12])		(teufelsdreck)	
70	agaricum (agaric[13])	holze schwame	*holzschwamm	Ventura 15 calidus est et siccus in secundo gradu. Cf. 6″ and Marzell.

9 Daems 32 has aspargus lŏchknúp, tentatively identified with *Allium cepa* L. (onion).

10 Ventura 509 does not give the degree of heat, as does the Hebrew, so it cannot be the source here (as, for instance, in 68). The German form with -s- and not -t- (English 'nettle') is distinctive for the area where the translation cannot have been produced.

11 The front vowel before *s impurum* (= s + consonant) is typical of the Romance area, cf. Mensching 78,1 espodio, the following entry 66, 80 and 108 below, and already above 45.

12 Here treated as one word (otherwise the gen. would be ase fetide), not yet attested.

13 agaric appears to be a vernacular form since it is not found in Latin dictionaries. Stirling lists a number of possible identifications, but not the fungus referred to here.

(*cont.*)

	Latin	German	Grimm	Notes
71	aloe hepaticum (aloe epatisi)			Stirling s.v. has *aloe* both as feminine and neuter.
72	aloe caballinum (aloe cabolini)			
72a	aloe citrinum			The three kinds are *aloe hepaticum, caballinum* and *citrinum* (Ventura 1 writes *cicotrinum*, which seems to be an error,[14] cf. Mensching 67,7).
73	*uncertain*	*uncertain*		
74	eruca (eruca)	gernol	gernol[15]	Grimm s.v.; cf. 12 above. Ventura 169 calida est et sicca in tertio gradu.
75	*uncertain*			
76	hepatica (epatisi[16])	leber krut	leberkraut	Daems 195.
77	epithymum (epitimi)			Daems 194. Ventura 159 calidum est et siccum in tertio gradu.
78	auellane (aleuanis[17])	gebrant hasel nus	haselnusz	Cf. 243 below. No degrees in Ventura 56.
79	[bolus] Armenicus (armenici[18])			Cf. 122 below and Ventura 60 frigidus est et siccus in secundo gradu.
80	scolopendria (ascolopendrie[19])	hirze zunge	hirschzunge	Daems 438. No degree given in Ventura 465.
81	hedera (edere)			gumma edere is mentioned in Ventura 172 and Daems 200 (also: sucus edere[20]). Cf. 94 below.
82	*uncertain*	*uncertain*		
83	*uncertain*	dorndistel	dorndistel	In Grimm and Marzell for several plants, unidentified.

14 But Daems 17 has succotrinum, for which see MLW s.v. aloe; but see DMLBS for cicotrinum s.v. aloe (b).

15 Probably the same as Daems 192 gerrole.

16 Impossible to decide whether the Hebrew stands for the genitive of epaticum or epatica.

17 Perhaps auellanas like Mensching 124,32 was intended.

18 Mensching 79,43 Armenium, id est bolo armenico, shows that bolus may be omitted.

19 For a-, see above on 65.

20 Daems: swart clibber dat uter ederen bomen loept (black goo that runs from the ivy tree).

(*cont.*)

	Latin	German	Grimm	Notes
83a		brakwurze	brachwurz	Daems 196*.
84	anthophyllum (antofili)	di gros wisenglokn	*grosze wiesenglocke	Cf. Daems 69 and Stirling. Grimm and Marzell only list 'wiesenglocke'.
85	... lapis (in epati lapis)			The Hebrew explanation suggests *in epati* (*hepate*) = in the liver.
86	*uncertain*	wilde magsame	wilder magsame	Cf. Daems 361.
87	*uncertain*	*uncertain*		
88	sputamentum (sputamentum)			
89	antimonium (antimonia[21])	zine esche	zainasche	Cf. Grimm s.v. zain (zainasche, zainesche must be burnt antimony). Ventura 13 calidum est et siccum in quarto gradu. Cf. 56.
90	*uncertain*	linin?	*linnen; leinen	
91	iua	*uncertain*		Ventura 242. uirtutem habet calidam et siccam in tertio gradu.
92	apronia?	*uncertain*		Cf. Stirling s.v. apronia.
93	*uncertain*			If the first word represents staphisagria (istafisagria[22]), it is not a gum; the Hebrew word means 'oleander'. Cf. 309.
94	hedera (edera)	gunde rebe	grundrebe	gundrebe is the older form, cf. Grimm s.v. grundrebe. No degrees given in Ventura 172.
95	iris (iris)	blaschwertel	blaue schwertel	Ventura 234 calidus est et siccus in secundo gradu, as in 17 above.
96	origanum (origino)	*winde		This meaning of 'winde' not in Grimm or Marzell.

21 For -ia, cf. DMLBS s.v. antimonium.

22 On i- or a-, see above at 65.

(*cont.*)

	Latin	German	Grimm	Notes
97	ebulus (ebulus)	atik	attich	Cf. 13 above.
98	inula campana (inula canpana)	alant	alant	Same degrees as in Ventura 160, cf. 4 above.
99	esula (esula)	wolvis milk	wolfsmilch	Ventura 168 calida est et sicca in quarto gradu. Daems 196. Cf. 10 above.
100	adianthus (adiantus)	*batonie (kleine)	batonie	Ventura 40 uirtutem habet calidam et humidam in primo gradu. The German word refers to Stachys officinalis and thus does not match.
101	*uncertain*	lebendik kalk	lebendiger kalk	The Latin must be a corrupt form of asbestus,[23] as in Ventura 123 Calx, albestix, alnestrion,[24] calcis uiua idem est. Calida est et sicca in tertio gradu. Cf. 181 below.
102	atriplex (antriplex[25])	melde	melde	Ventura 47 frigidum est in primo gradu, humidum in secundo.
103	amygdala (amigdelarum)			Ventura 24 calide sunt et sicce in secundo gradu.
103a	amygdala amara (amigdalarum amararum)			
104	*uncertain*	neslin same	nesselsame	Daems 468 netelsat.[26]
105	anabulla (anabula)	berin krut	*bärenkraut	Daems 29; Marzell s.v. bärenkraut and beerenkraut refers to different plants; cf. 112 below.

23 ἡ ἄσβεστος 'unslaked lime, quicklime'; Mensching 73,41 Alpeton, id est albestion (albeston M), id est cal biua; 64,1 Aueston es cal biua, cf. MLW s.v. asbestus, DMLBS s.v. asbestos, reading אסבישטוש.

24 Read: aluestrion.

25 For an example of an-, see DMLBS s.v. atriplex.

26 A79 achantis, urtica purgens in García González must of course read urtica pungens, with Daems 468, which is what Mowat had printed, see DMLBS s.v. urtica. (purgens is not Latin; the participle of purgo is purgans.)

(*cont.*)

	Latin	German	Grimm	Notes
106	anacocci? (anacodi)	wakolder ber	wacholder-beeren	A235 anacochi, Daems 629 is bay berries (bakeler), not juniper berries.
107	arnoglossa (arnoglosa)	wegbreid	weg(e)breit	Daems 5.
108	scoria (iscorion[27])			
109	anthera (antera)	rosen same	rosensame	Daems 27. Cf. MLW s.v. anthera 2). Ventura 49 semen quod reperitur in medio rosarum.[28]
110	eupatorium (enpatorium[29])	wilde salbe	wildsalbei	Cf. 1 above.
111	*uncertain*	bivenele	bibenelle	armoracia is not attested as a synonym of pimpinella; cf. 114 and Daems 372.
112	*uncertain*	bere krut	bärenkraut	Many plants, cf. Marzell and 105 above.
113	agrimonia (argimonia)	eberwurzen	eberwurz	Marzell s.v.; cf. 248 below.
114	armoracia (armorica)	heiderik	heiderich, hederich	See MLW s.v. armoracia 2).
115	*uncertain*	gundrum	gundram, gundelrebe	Cf. Grimm s.v. grundrebe and 94 above.
116	atrapassa (atropasta)	holderblumen	holunderblüte	Stirling s.v. Daems 425*.
117	arcontilla (arcontila)	kazen zagel	katzenzagel	Daems 179 and 424.
118	balsamita (balsamita)	bruke minze	*bruchminze	Grimm, Daems and Marzell have only 'bachminze'; Mentha aquatica (also called wasserminze).
119	balsamum (balsama)	balsame	balsam	

27 On isc-, see 65 above.

28 This can be seen clearly on the illustration of Ms London, British Library, Egerton 747, fol. 11r, which is online (http://www.bl.uk/manuscripts/Viewer.aspx?ref=egerton_ms_747_fs001r#).

29 The spelling en- instead of eu- not noted in DMLBS or MLW, but Ventura 162 n. 1 quotes it from Herbarijs (Middle Dutch).

(*cont.*)

	Latin	German	Grimm	Notes
120	bacca lauri (*baclor)	lorber	lorbeer	
121	blacte Byzantie[30] (blacte bisanzie)	*fische aug	fischauge	Cf. MLW s.v. 2. blatta, Ventura 86 est autem blacte biçantie oculus quedam(!) piscium similis limaccia, and B44.
122	bolus Armenicus (boli arminisi[31])			Cf. 79 above and 140 below.
123	bryonia (brionie)	wilde kurb(is)	wildkürbis	Cf. Marzell and Daems 82 (hundeskürbis).
124	portulaca (bortulace)	wurze	*wurz	Daems 357 wurczeln. Grimm s.v. sauwurz 5); cf. Grimm s.v. wurz 2) b) γ).
125	*uncertain*			
126	*uncertain*	hagen apel	hagapfel	Cf. Daems 98 bedagar[32] hagenopfel; Marzell identifies hagenapfel with Crataegus oxyacanthus.
127	penidia (benidit[33])			Daems 389 penidium, Grimm s.v. benetzucker and zuckerbenet; Engl. pennet.
128	branca ursina (branca ursina)	beren kluen	bärenklau	Daems 95. Ventura 67 calida est et humida in primo gradu.
129	balaustia (balustie[s])	granat opel blut	granatapfelblüte	Ventura 61 frigida est et sicca in secundo gradu.
130	bardana (bardana)	hufe latik	huflattich	Daems 85. Cf. Stirling s.v. bardana.
131	bdellium (bdeli)			Ventura 80 calidum est in secundo gradu, humidum in primo.

30 K.S. Moosmann, *Tierische Drogen im 18. Jahrhundert im Spiegel offizineller und nicht offizineller Literatur und ihre Bedeutung für die Gegenwart*, Stuttgart 2019 (Quellen und Studien zur Geschichte der Pharmazie, vol. 119), 248–252.

31 One of the few cases where Latin -ci is rendered as -si.

32 Ventura 79 bedeguard, id est spina alba, frigida est in primo gradu. B31 bedegar, rubus idem. MLW s.v. bedegar. Lexer s.v. hagenaphel has spinella (see Stirling s.v.) as equivalent.

33 The form in -t possibly influenced by benedictus, past participle of benedico, ere; cf. Lexer s.v. benît.

(*cont.*)

	Latin	German	Grimm	Notes
132	*uncertain*			
133	borago (boraginis)	burs blumin	bauern-blume	Cf. Marzell s.v. 'bauernblume' and 'bauernborretsch'.
134	ballota[34] (balota)	andorn	andorn	Daems 648. Again at 155, 209 and 291 below.
135	*beata[35] (beata)	iserin herz	eisenherz	Daems 471.
136	basilia (basilia)	muter wurz[36]	mutterwurz	Cf. Daems 350, 429 and 90* and Marzell s.v. for various other plants.
137	basilicus (basilicus)	muter krut	mutterkraut	Cf. Grimm and Marzell s.v., many different plants, and MLW s.v. 3. basilicus.
138	buglossa (buglosa)	oksin (okson) zunge	ochsenzunge	
139	brathy (*brecdeos)	seven bom	sevenbaum	Daems 416 and 416* bracteos[37], MLW s.v. bratheos. Cf. 258 and 25″.
140	bolus (bolus)	blutstain	*blutstein[38]	Cf. 79 and 122 above, Ventura 60 contra … sanguinis fluxum.
141	basilicum (basilicum)	basilie	basilie	Marzell s.v., cf. 19 above.
142	bruscus (bruscus)	stain breke	steinbrech	Daems 103.
143	caryophyllon (garofali)	nelikin[39]	nelke	Ventura 200 gariofili calidi et sicci in tertio gradu.
144	[galgan]		galgan	Again, like in 16 above, the lemma is a German form for Latin galanga.
145	galbanum (galbanum)	galgan	galgan	Ventura 203 calidum est in tertio gradu, humidum in primo. Cf. Grimm s.v. galban and galgan 3c).

34 MLW and DMLBS s.v. ballote.
35 Stirling refers from beata to beta, no lemma in MLW or DMLBS.
36 Cf. metewrz MLW s.v. basilia, metwurcz Daems 350, perhaps confused by the translator or the copyist.
37 In 121 above (blacta), -ct- represented a Romance spelling equivalent to Latin -tt-; *brecdeos for bracteos = brateos shows, that this could be realized as -c-, i.e. /k/.
38 Grimm and Daems 299 have this word only as translation of lapis haematites.
39 See Grimm s.v. nägelchen for MHG forms.

(*cont.*)

	Latin	German	Grimm	Notes
146	granum paradisi (grani paradisi)	pardis korner	paradies-körner	Cf. Grimm s.v.; a different plant in Marzell s.v. paradieskorn.
147	*perhaps* gallia mus-cata (galia muscade)			Cf. DMLBS s.v. gallia.
148	git	raden	raden	Cf. 164.
149	gelena (gelena)	toste	dost	Daems 343. Cf. Stirling.
150	gerontea (gerontea)	swerdel	schwertel	Daems 235.
151	tragacanthum (draganti)			Ventura 152 frigidum est in secundo gradu, humidum in primo.
152	*uncertain*	wilde fenkel	wilder fenchel	Daems 207 and 364.
153	ossa dactylorum (dactilorum)	daitel kern	dattelkern	-ai- in daitel is without parallel. Cf. 128″.
154	diagridium[40] (dia-gridi)	s⟨k⟩ameni	skammonie	Ventura 151 calidum est et siccum in quarto gradu.
155	*uncertain*	andorn	andorn	Cf. 134, 209 and 291.
156	uiola (uiolarum)	violen	viole	Daems 469. Ventura 504 frigida est in primo gradu, humida in fine secundi gradi(!).
156a	filipendula (vilipen-dola)			Cf. Ventura 180.
157	uirga pastoris (wirga pastori)	hirtenstaf	hirtenstab	
158	tithymallus (titimali)			Cf. 160 below.

40 Greek δακρύδιον 'tear' (applied to the juice of scammony) was confused with drug names starting with δια- 'containing', and the corrupt form became standard in Latin texts from late antiquity onwards, cf. J. Svennung, *Wortstudien zu den spätlateinischen Oribasius-rezensionen*, Uppsala 1933 (Uppsala Universitets Årsskrift, vol. 5), 73–74, C.T. Lewis and Ch. Short, *A Latin Dictionary*, Oxford 1880 (online at https://logeion.uchicago.edu/), s.v. diagrydium, Stirling s.v. diagridium and dacrydion; surprisingly, there is no entry in André. Diosc. *mat. med.* 4.170.1 describes the collection of the juice of σκαμμωνία; the synonym δακρύδιον is a later addition in the codices RV of Dioscorides; it is found (as *diagridium*) in Galen. *alfab.* 252, as is κολοφώνιουμ.

(*cont.*)

	Latin	German	Grimm	Notes
159	terebinthina (terebentina)	luter harz	lauteres harz	Grimm only lists 'flieszharz'; cf. Grimm s.v. lauter 18).
160	tithymallus (titimali)	zwickele	zwickel	Cf. 158; Marzell only for other plants.
161	thapsia? (tapsia)			
162	iusquiamus (iusquiami)	bilse same	bilsensame	Ventura 231 frigide complexionis est in tertio gradu, siccum in secundo.
163	gentiana (jinzine)	enzion	enzian	Above 14. As in 164, the first letter of the Latin word is taken to represent g-, which in some dialects may be pronounced j-, likewise in 165.
164	git (jit)	rade	raden	Cf. 148 above. Ventura 206 calida est et sicca in secundo gradu.
165	gingiber (jinjiberi)	ingeber	ingwer	Daems 486*. Ventura 518 calidum est in tertio gradu, humidum in secundo.
166	iuniperus (iuniperi)	wekolter ber	wacholderbeere	
167	*uncertain*	tob wurze	taubwurz?	'taubwurz' is a synonym of aristolochia in N.I. Annenkov, *Botanisches Wörterbuch oder Sammlung der Namen*[41] ..., Moskva 1876, and cf. Grimm s.v. hohlwurz and taub 6) a).
168	lactuca (lactuse)	latik	lattich	Ventura 257 temperate frigida est et humida.
169	lignum aloes (lignum aloes)	himel holze	*himmelholz	Ventura 2 calidum est et siccum in secundo gradu.
170	lingua ceruina (lingua ceruine)	hirz zunge	hirschzunge	Cf. 280a below.

41 Botaničeskij slovar' ili sobranie nazvanij kak russkich tak imnogich inostrannych rastenij na jazykach latinskom, russkom, némezkom ...

(*cont.*)

	Latin	German	Grimm	Notes
171	lingua auis (lingua auis)	vogel zunge	vogelzunge	Cf. Grimm s.v. vogelzunge 3).
172	leuisticum (leuisticum)	liber stikel	liebstöckel	Ventura 266 calidus est et siccus in secundo gradu.
173	lupinus (lupinus)	wike bone	wickenbohne	Daems 617, and cf. Grimm s.v. wickenstroh.
174	laureola (lavreola)	sprink korner	springkörner[42]	Cf. Marzell s.v. springkorn; here, Daphne mezereum is probably meant. Cf. 199 below.
175	*uncertain*	zigen bek	ziegenbock	Cf. Marzell s.v.
176	lithargyrum (litarjirum)	golt esche	goldasche	Grimm s.v. goldstein 5). Ventura 255 temperatum est in frigiditate et siccitate.
177	lapis haematites (lapis ematites)	blutstain	blutstein	Daems 299.
178	*uncertain*			Since no medical use of the tree laburnum seems to be attested, perhaps libanum (incense) or labdanum, below 190.
179	liquiricia; glycyrrhiza (lacrize)	lakriz	lakritze	Ventura 248 temperate calida est et humida.
180	lapis calaminaris (lapis calaminaris)	kalemin stain	galmei	Daems 281. Cf. Grimm s.v. galmei 2) a).
181	lapis calcis[43] (lapis calcis)	kalk stain	kalkstein	Here, 'quicklime' (calx uiua) is meant. Cf. 101.
182	lapis lyncis (lapis lincis)	wolf stain	*wolf(s)stein	Ventura 296.[44] Another mineral in Grimm s.v. wolf G. 4).

42 A different plant Daems 158.

43 The Latin expression here may well result from a confusion with chalcus, see MLW s.v. 2. calx, C. 'hot in the fourth degree' can only be said of quicklime.

44 Not in Goltz. It seems rather to belong to the sphere of magic and is mentioned in lapidaries, e.g. Euax-Damigeron ch. 43, and Marbode, but also in Rufinus.

(*cont.*)

	Latin	German	Grimm	Notes
183	*uncertain*	kers same	*kirschsame (= kirsch-kern)	
184	limatura auri (limature auri)	gesegint golt	goldstaub	Cf. Grimm s.v. goldstaub 2) and Ventura 3.
185	lenticula[45] (lenticula)	linsin	linse	Ventura 263 frigide et sicce complexionis est.
186	lapis agapis (lapis agapis)	beril	beryll	L35; Ventura 268; cf. Grimm s.v. brill (but the lapis agapis is not a precious stone). MLW s.v. agapis, DMLBS s.v. achates 2c.
187	labrum Veneris (labrum ueneris)	gros tistele	grosze distel	Cf. Grimm s.v. distel 1) and große distel in Marzell.
188	lathyris, latirida (lactirida)	spine wurz	spinnenwurz	Cf. Grimm s.v.
189	elelisphacus (lelifagus)	salbaie	salbei	
190	laudanum (labdanum)			
191	lilium (lilium)	lilien	lilie	Ventura 250 calidum est et humidum.
192	lapis lazuli (lapis lasuli)	lazur	lasurstein	Ventura 249 frigide et sicce complexionis est.
193	linum (linis[46])	line	leinen	Cf. Grimm s.v. leinen n. Ventura 277 calida est et humida. Cf. 256.
194	lycium (licium)			Ventura 253 calidum est in primo gradu, siccum in secundo.
195	lapathium (lapacium)	kletten krut	klettenkraut	Daems 285.
196	*uncertain*			

45 Daems 297 lenticula wasserlinsi, more likely meant here than the food.
46 The s in linis may best be explained as an abbreviation of semen (seed), i.e., linseed.

(*cont.*)

	Latin	German	Grimm	Notes
197	laurus (laurus)	lorberen bom	lorbeerbaum	
198	lentiscus (lentiscus)	*uncertain*		Ventura 262 calide et sicce complexionis est.
199	laureola (laureola)	sprink korner	springkörner	Cf. 174 above.
200	*uncertain*[47]			
201	lapis Armenicus (lapis armenicus)			Same as lapis lazuli in Ventura 270.
202	lapis pyrites (lapis piricis)	vur stain	feuerstein	
203	mastix (mastisis[48])	mastik	mastix	Ventura 294 calida est et sicca in secundo gradu.
204	milium solis (milium solis)	stain breche	steinbrech	Daems 334 and 635; cf. 278 and 317. Ventura 207 granum solis calidum est et siccum in tertio gradu.
205	mandragora (mandragora)	alrune	alraun	Ventura 300 frigida est et sicca.
206	margarita (margaritarum)	perlin	perle	Ventura 298 frigida est et sicca.
207	macis (macis)	muskaden blumen	muskatblume	Ventura 310 calida est et sicca in secundo gradu.
208	marathrum (maretri)	venchel same	fenchelsame	Ventura 182 feniculus calidus est et siccus in secundo gradu. Cf. 228 and 292 below.
209	marrubium (marubiu⟨m⟩)	andorn	andorn	Ventura 305 calidum est et siccum in tertio gradu. Cf. 291 below.
210	mumia (mumia)	toden flaisch	totenfleisch	Ventura 299 calida est et sicca in quarto gradu.
211	*uncertain*	*baldrion	baldrian	Cf. 297.

47 lactapucia instead of catapucia?
48 Another case of סי for -ci-.

(*cont.*)

	Latin	German	Grimm	Notes
212	*uncertain*[49]	somer opel	sommerapfel	Cf. Marzell s.v., where the German word means melon.[50] Cf. also 260 below.
213	muscus (musci)	bisame	bisam	Daems 310. Ventura 308 calidus est et siccus in secundo gradu.
214	*uncertain*	wilde petersilie	wilde petersilie	Refers to various plants in Marzell. Ventura 359 calidum est et siccum in secundo gradu.
215	melilotum (melilotum)	kunigs krone	königskrone	M8 mellilotum herba est cuius semen dicitur corona regia.
216	myrtilli (mirtili)	haidelber	heidelbeere	Ventura 288 frigida est in primo gradu, sicca in secundo.
217	morum (morum)	branber[51]	brombeere	Ventura 315 calidi sunt et sicci. Daems 325; cf. 223.
218	morum (mora)	mulber	maulbeere	Daems 331.
219	*uncertain*[52]	milde	melde	
220	malua (malua)	papel	pappel	Daems 631. Ventura 291 frigida est et humida in secundo gradu.
220a	bismalua (bis malua)	ibisch	eibisch	Daems 99. Ventura 292 calidus est et humidus in secundo gradu.[53]
221	*uncertain*			For asa fetida (teufelsdreck), cf. 69 above, different from melissa (melisa).
222	*uncertain*	*uncertain*		The first word may hide the second part, marini, of a plant name; the German could be bomekin = bäumchen.
223	*morum ribesi (morum ribesi)	*bronber	brombeere	Unusual expression for red or black currant. Cf. 217?

49 milinci could be the gen. of melanthium.
50 One could emend the Hebrew, but melons are cold and moist.
51 Definitely not to be interpreted as braunbeere; for the form, cf. Grimm s.v. brombeere.
52 melonis (i.e., melon) would at least be cold.
53 Ventura 293 is also bismalua (malua ortensis, quod alii uocant bismalua).

(*cont.*)

	Latin	German	Grimm	Notes
224	melissa (melisa)	metere	meter	Cf. Grimm s.v. meter f. 2) and Marzell s.v. metere.
225	maurella (morela)	nahtschatte	nachtschatten	Daems 306. Cf. 275.
226	memitha (memita)	schelle wurz	schellwurz	Daems 115.
227	*uncertain*	*uncertain*		
228	marathrum (maratrum)	venchel	fenchel	The German equivalent never has w-, so וו must render the letter v- = /f/; cf. 208 and 292.
229	*uncertain*	*uncertain*		
230	myrobalani (mirobalani)			
230a	Citrini (citrini)			See Ventura 309 and M4 for five kinds of *myrobalanus*.
230b	Indi (indi)			
230c	bellirici (bilareci)			Cf. Engl. belleric.
230d	emblici (emlisi[54])			
230e	kebuli (kebuli)			
230f		laxiren	laxieren	Cf. 354a.
231	*uncertain*			
231a	*uncertain*	*uncertain*		The German is very similar to the equally unexplained word in 222 above.
232	manna (mana)	himels brot	himmelsbrot	Grimm s.v. 1).
233	nigella (nijela)	radin	raden	Cf. 164 above and Grimm s.v.
234	neprus? (nepre)	kle blumin	*kleeblumen	Various identifications in Grimm and Marzell; for nepra, cf. Daems 335*.
235	nux (nucis + *uncertain*)	wilit nus	*wilde nusz?	
236	nux muscata (nucis muscade)	muskat nuse	muskatnusz	Cf. 242 below.

54 Another case of סי for -ci.

(*cont.*)

	Latin	German	Grimm	Notes
237	nardostachys (nardostacios)			
237a	nardus Indica (nardus indica)			
237b	spica nardi (spica nardi)			Could also be German (spikenarde), but cf. 237a and 344.
238	nardus Celtica (nardus celtica)			
238a	spica Celtica (spica celtica)			
239	napy (napi)	senf same	senfsame	νᾶπυ; cf. 272 below.
240	nardelaeon (nardileon)			ναρδέλαιον.
241	nepeta (nepeta)	minte	minze	
242	nux myristica (nux miristica)	muskat nuse	muskatnusz	Cf. 236 above.
243	nux Pontica (nux pontica)	hasel nuse	haselnusz	Cf. 78 above.
244	storax (storax)			
244a	storax calamita (storax calamite)			Cf. 245.
244b	storax rubea (rubea)			
244c	storax confita (storax comfita)			
244d	cozymbrum (cozimbrum)			S46 ... dicunt quidam quod calamite fex est rubea ... et confite fex cozimbrum, confita idem est quod thimiama. Cf. MLW s.v. cozumbrum and DMLBS s.v. cozumber.
245	storax calamita (storacis calamente[55])	stik narde		For 'stik', cf. Grimm s.v. storax 2); 'narde' = storax is not attested, but both are used for perfumes.

55 For -nt-, see MLW s.v. calamites.

(*cont.*)

	Latin	German	Grimm	Notes
246	*uncertain*	wilde kume	*wilder kümmel	kume = kümmel Grimm s.v. kümmel I 4) b).
247	sil montanum (sili monteni)	grose same	grossame	A different plant in Marzell s.v. grossame.
248	*uncertain*	eber wurze	eberwurz	Cf. 113 above.
249	sulfur (sulfur)	swebel	schwefel	Ventura 422 calidum est et siccum in primo gradu.
250	spica (spise)	wilde spik	wilde spiek	
251	xylobalsamum (silobalsami)			Cf. 340 below.
252	saluia (saluia)	selbe	salbei	Ventura 447 calida est in primo gradu, sicca in secundo.
253	citrinum (sitrinum)			Perhaps the same as pomum citrinum.[56]
254	sambucus (sanpuci)	holunder	holunder	Ventura 453 calidus est in secundo gradu, siccus in primo. See 338 below.
255	sambacus[57] (sanbocus)	holunder	holunder	Ventura 472 ex floribus fit oleum sambacinum.
255a	sambacinum (sanbocinum)			sambacinum (oleum)
256	semen lini (semen lini)	line same	leinsame	Cf. 193 above.
257	*uncertain*			
258	sabina (sabina)	saven bom	sabenbaum	Ventura 441 calida est et sicca in tertio gradu. Cf. 139 above and 25″.
259	struthium (strucium)	wilde kol	wilder kohl	Daems 734. Cf. Ventura 436 n. 1.
260	citrullus (citruli)	somer opel	sommerapfel	Daems 159*. Ventura 118. Cf. 212 above and 328, and Grimm s.v. erdapfel.

56 Since it grows on a tree, Daems 179* is not a possible match.

57 DMLBS does not distinguish between sambucus and sambacus.

(*cont.*)

	Latin	German	Grimm	Notes
261	sanguis draconis (sanguis draconis)			S5 sanguis draconis succus est cuiusdam herbe, non sanguis, ut quidam mentiuntur. Ventura 425.
262	*uncertain*	*uncertain*		
263	sal communis (salis comunis)			Mensching 152,42.
264	sal nitri (sal nitri)			
265	fenum[58] Graecum (fenogrecum)	krisch howe	griechisch heu	
266	squilla (squila)	mer zwibil	meerzwiebel	Cf. 66 above.
267	sumach (sumac)			Ventura 456[59] frigidum est in secundo gradu, siccum in tertio. Virtutem habet constringendi.
268	spodium (spodium)	gebrant helfenbain	gebranntes elfenbein	
268a		galgen	galgan	Grimm s.v. galgan, not mentioned in this connection in other sources.
268b	semen bombycis (semen bonbacis)	baumwole same	baumwoll-samen	
269	sucus liquoricie (sucus licorice)			
270	serapinum (sera-pinum[60])			
270a	sagapenum (saga-pinum)			-pen- and -pin- are both current.
271	sarcocolla (sar-cocola)			S10 gumma est, et interpretatur glutinum ad carnem. Ventura 428 calida est et sicca in quarto gradu.
271a	glutinum (glutinum)			
272	sinapi (sinapi)	senf	senf	Cf. 239 above.

58 Mistaking f- for s- (ſ) can only occur in a Latin manuscript, and with a copyist who does not know the meaning of fenum.

59 A229 is something else.

60 serapina not attested so far.

(*cont.*)

	Latin	German	Grimm	Notes
273	cinnamomum (sinamomi)	kanele	kanel	Grimm s.v. claims this for Low German and the Rhineland.
274	semperuiuum (semparwifum)	hus wirze	hauswurz	Ventura 421 Virtutem habent frigidam in tertio gradu, siccam in primo.
275	solatrum (soletero)	nacht schade	nachtschatte	Daems 718. Cf. Grimm s.v. nachtschatte 3) and 225.
276	squinantum (squinantum)			Cf. 45 above.
276a	palea camelorum (palea camalarum)			
277	*uncertain*			
278	saxifraga (saxifrija[61])	stain breche	steinbrech	Cf. 204 and 317.
279	sinonum (sinanum)			S68. Daems 365 and 665.
279a	petroselinum agreste (petarselinum agreste)	wilde petersilie	wilde petersilie	Cf. 214 above.
280	sandaraca (sandaraca)			S79 sandaraca id est auripigmentum rubeum.
280a	auripigmentum rubeum (auripicmanetum rubeum)			
281	scolopendria (scolependiria)			S89 scolopendria lingua ceruina idem.
281a	lingua ceruina (lingua ceruena)	hirz zunge	hirschzunge	Cf. 170 above.
282	smireos (smireos)			Cf. S116 (with app. crit.), 120″ below and DMLBS s.v. smyrnium: smirtus (read: smirius) est betonica *SB* (*Sinonoma Bartholomei*) 40?[62]
282a	betonica (betonica)	betonie	betonie	

61 It is also possible to read saxifrigia, see DMLBS s.v. saxifragus. Stirling also has saxifragia.

62 Stirling s.v. (s)myrrhis is another plant. Stirling may be mistaken in referring from smirnus to myrtus.

(*cont.*)

	Latin	German	Grimm	Notes
283	ambra (ambra)			Ventura 29 ambra calida est et sicca in secundo gradu … dicitur esse sperma ceti (cete, id est balene).
283a	balene (balene)			
284	peganum (pegani)	wilde rute	wilde raute	Daems 386. Cf. 321.
285	folium (folii)	negelken bleter	nelkenblätter	F25 folium quando simpliciter ponitur pro foliis gariofilorum intellegitur.[63]
286	piper longum (piper lonji)	lange peper	langer pfeffer	Ventura 355 piper calidum est in principio quarti gradi(!), siccum in medio.
287	petroselinum (petroselini)	petersilie	petersilie	Ventura 359 calidum est et siccum in secundo gradu.
288	pyrethrum (piritrum)	berchtram	berchtram	Ventura 354 calidum est et siccum in tertio gradu. Cf. 314 below.
289	peganum (pegani)	stab wirze	*stabwurz	Ventura 407. Daems, Grimm and Marzell refer to other plants.
290	*palea (palea)	garwe	garbe	Daems 316. No other attestation for palea = Achillea millefolium.[64]
291	prasium (prasii)	andorn	andorn	Cf. 134, 155 and 209.
292	feniculum (feniculi)	venchel	fenchel	Cf. 208 and 228 above.
293	beryllus (perili)	beril	brill	Cf. Mensching 124,9.
293a		kristal	kristall	
294	polytrichum (politricum)	nise wurze	nieswurz	Daems 382.
295	*folium citrinum (folii citrini)	gele lilien	gelbe lilie	For other plants cf. Daems and Marzell. The Latin does not seem to be attested; error folium instead of lilium at some point?

63 Same interpretation in Mensching 111,4, probably incorrect, since it does not occur in other sources, see André and Stirling s.v. folium.

64 Nevertheless, Grimm s.v. haberstroh refers to garbe.

(*cont.*)

	Latin	German	Grimm	Notes
296	petroleum (petrolii)			The Hebrew explanation is for chrism ('holy oil'), associated with St Peter (Peter's oil) and Rome, not found in other sources.
297	phu (fu)	*baldrion	baldrian	Ventura 179 calidum est et siccum in secundo gradu. Daems 220. Cf. 211.
298	peonia (peonia)	begonien korner	*päonienkörner	Ventura 356 calida est et sicca in secundo gradu. 'korner' must refer to the seeds, cf. Grimm s.v. gichtkorn.
299	pinum (pinum)	tan apel	tannapfel	Should be recognised as a separate lemma different from pinus, i, cf. Grimm.
300	prunum (prunum)	praumen	pflaumen	Ventura 362 frigida sunt et humida.
301	pix naualis (pix naualis)	pech von schifen	pech von schiffen	Ventura 378 calida et sicca in secundo gradu.
302	polypodium (polipodium)	*uncertain*		
303	peucedanum (peucedani)	wild fenchel	wilder fenchel	Cf. Ventura 358 n. 1, Marzell and Grimm s.v. saufenchel.
304	pomum citrinum (pomi sitrini)			Ventura 372 cortex … calida est et sicca, interior substantia frigida et sicca.
305	fumus terre (fumi terre)	toben krop	taubenkropf	Ventura 178 calidus est in primo gradu, siccus in secundo. Same as 306.
305a	*uncertain*			
306	fumitera (fumitera)	ert rute	erdraute	Cf. DMLBS s.v. 1 fumus 4) and 305 above. Grimm s.v.
307	pilosella (pilosela)	muse ore	mausohr	Grimm s.v. mäuseohr 3).
308	flammula (flamula)			F20 flammula est herba calida et sicca in quarto gradu, masticata exurit linguam sicut ignis. Ventura 176.

(*cont.*)

	Latin	German	Grimm	Notes
309	stafisagria (fisagra)	*uncertain*		Ventura 457 calida est et sicca in tertio gradu. Daems 443 staphisagra; cf. DMLBS and Stirling s.v. staphis. Cf. 93 above?
310	plantago (plantaginis)	wegerich	wegerich	
311	pistacee (pistacearum)	hasel nus	haselnusz	Ventura 375 similes pineis.
312	pinee (pinearum)	welsche nus	wälsche nusz[65]	Ventura 361 calida est et humida.
313	puleium (puleium)	puleie	polei	Ventura 369 calidum est et siccum in tertio gradu.
314	pyrethrum (pireticum)	berchtram	berchtram	Cf. 288 above.
315	parietaria (paritaria)	nacht un tak	nacht und tag	Daems 366; Grimm and Marzell record this for tag und nacht.
316	potentilla (portentila[66])	grensink	grensing	Grimm s.v. 1) a).
317	polytrichum (politricum)	stain breche	*steinbrech	This identification not in Grimm or Marzell. Cf. 204 and 278.
318	pastinaca (pastinaca)	morchen	möhre	
319	*uncertain*	agermunde	agermund	Perhaps agrimonia aprella Daems 490.
320	papyrus (popirus)	bisen	binse	Daems 272*.
321	peganum (peganum)	wilt ruten	wilde raute	Cf. 284.
322	pipinella (pipinela)	bivenele	bibenelle	
323	cinnamomum (cinamomi[67])	cinamin	zimt	Cf. Grimm s.v. zimt.
324	zeduarium (zeduari)	zidwan	zitwer	Daems 485.

65 Walnuts, error for pine nuts.

66 For port-, see DMLBS s.v. potentilla.

67 The Hebrew spelling is hard to explain, ps- would be easier, cf. 156″ psidia = σίδια.

(*cont.*)

	Latin	German	Grimm	Notes
325	cyclamen (ciclamen)	schwins brot	schweinsbrot	
326	*uncertain*	*uncertain* + kerne		
327	cyperus (ciperi)	wilde galgan	wilder galgan	Grimm s.v. galgan 1) b). Ventura 110 calidus et siccus in secundo gradu.
328	citrullus (citruli)	erd apel	erdapfel	Daems 159*. Cf. Grimm s.v. and 260 above.
329	centaurea (centaurea)			Ventura 96. Daems 111 and 538. Cf. Mensching 93,10.
330	cerussa[68] (cerusa)	bli esche	bleiasche	Error for 'bleiweisz'?
331	cepe (cepe)	zwiboln	zwiebeln (plur.)	
332	*uncertain*	*uncertain*		
333	chaerophyllum (cerefolium)	kerbel	kerbel	
334	cinimum (cinimum)	kumel	kümmel	Daems 117. DMLBS s.v. cyminum for the alternative form cinimum.
335	chelidonia (celidonia)	schel wurz	schellwurz	
336	*uncertain*	wilde kumel	wildkümmel	The Latin is perhaps cerni, Grimm s.v. wildkümmel only quotes carni; feldkümmel is also possible, and cf. Marzell.
337	citrum (citrum)	jiden epel	judenapfel	
338	*uncertain*			
338a	sambucus (sambuci)	holunder	holunder	Cf. 254.
339	cichorium (cicori)	wege wise	wegeweise	
340	carpobalsamum (carpobalsami)	holz von balsam		Cf. Grimm s.v. fruchtbalsam and holzbalsam.
341	cassia lignea (casia lignea)	wilde zinamin	wilder zimt	

68 MLW s.v. cerussa 3c lists bliybeyse. See also Grimm s.v. bleiasche (= molybditis). Surprisingly, not in Daems.

(*cont.*)

	Latin	German	Grimm	Notes
342	cuscuta (cuscuta)	wilde siden	wilde seide	Ventura 91 calidum est in primo gradu, siccum in secundo. Daems 137; Grimm s.v. side and 360 below.
342a	reubarbarum (rebarba[69])			Cf. 378 below.
343	calamintha (calaminta)	spik narde	spikenarde	Not equivalent in Grimm or Marzell. Cf. 237b and 376.
344	cardamomum (cardamomi)			Ventura 92 calidum est et siccum in secundo gradu.
345	castoreum (castorei)	biber gaile[70]	bibergeil	Ventura 98 calidum est in tertio gradu, siccum in secundo.
346	chamaedrys (camedrios)	gamander	gamander	Ventura 103 calidum est et siccum in tertio gradu.
347	calamus aromaticus (calami aromatici)	merhelm	*meerhalm	Ventura 111 calidum est et siccum in secundo gradu.
348	caruum (carui)	wise kumel	weiszkümmel[71]	Ventura 105 carui calida est et sicca in tertio gradu. Daems 157.
349	crocus (croci)	garten safron	gartensafran	
350	cassia fistula (casia fistula)			Ventura 90 calida est et humida infra omnem gradum.
351	camphora (canfore)			Ventura 88 frigida est et sicca in tertio gradu.
352	Corycius (coricii)	schlote von spinel sam	schote des *spinell-samens?	The German is uncertain; Corycius (not in MLW and DMLBS) is a variety of saffron and does not fit the German.
352a	Cnidius (nidi)			Doubtful; usually part of coccus Cnidius, cf. 355.

69 For a shortened form, probably current and not just an error, see DMLBS s.v. reubarbarum and Mensching 143,16.

70 This may be the female noun (singular), or a form of the plural.

71 Wiesenkümmel is also possible, cf. Daems 157.

(*cont.*)

	Latin	German	Grimm	Notes
353	Creticus (cretisi[72])	figen?	feigen?	352, 352a and 353 are all adjectives of place-names.
354	colocynthis (colo-quintidis)	mer opel	meerapfel	Marzell has the German word only for Solanum tuberosum.
354a		laxatif	laxativ	Cf. 230f.
355	coccus Cnidius (coc nidi)	sprink wurz same	springwurz-same	Daems 169. The German word is, however, applied to a number of species; cf. 365.
356	cucurbita (cucur-bita)	kurbis	kürbis	Ventura 118.
357	colofonia (colofonia)	krischpech	griechisches pech	Grimm s.v. griechisch 3).
358	camomilla (camom-ila)			Cf. 371.
359	caro leonis (cornu leonis)			cornu 'horn' is an error.[73]
360	cuscuta (cuscute)	*uncertain*		Cf. 342.
361	cyperus (ciperus)	rote kol gros	*rotes kohl-gras	Not attested. (colgras Daems 525)
362	chamaepitys (camepiteos)	gamandre di gros	groszer gamander	Ventura 104 calidum est et siccum in tertio gradu. Grimm s.v. gaman-der 1) a) b).
363	cubebe (cubebis)			
364	coriandrum (cori-andri)			
365	cataputia (catapu-cia)	sprink wurze	springwurz	Cf. 355.
366	capillus Veneris (capili ueneris)	stain ⟨rut⟩	steinraute	Daems 156 capillus Veneris stein rut; Grimm s.v. steinraute 3).
367	consolida (consolda)	wal ⟨wurz⟩ di gros	grosze wall-wurz	Daems 129.

72 Error for carice, Ventura 196, Daems 178 and C49, a particular kind of figs?
73 This item of materia medica not in Daems or Ventura.

(*cont.*)

	Latin	German	Grimm	Notes
368	cardus benedictus (cardus benedictus)	sturz wurze[74]	*sturzwurz	Daems 165. Cf. 110a″.
369	crassula (crasula)	drus wurze	trüswurz	Daems 541a.
370	cotula fetida (cotula fetida)	hunds wurze blumen	*hundswurzblume	
371	*uncertain*	hunds + *uncertain*		Daems 164 cinoglossa hundeszung?
372	camomilla (camomila)	mai blumen	*maiblume	Marzell only for other species. Cf. 358 above.
373	*uncertain*	*uncertain*		
374	columbaria (columbaria)	stern wurze	*sternwurz	Other plants in Grimm and Marzell.
375	calendula (calendula)	ringel krut	ringelkraut	Grimm s.v. ringelblume.
376	calamentum (calamentum)	stain minze	steinminze	Grimm s.v. steinminze 2). Cf. 343 above.
377	cardamonium (cardamonium)	wilde kres	wildkresse	cardamonium (cardamomum) is here, and indeed often, confused with cardamum, cf. MLW s.v. cardamomum 2a.
378	chalcanthum (calcantum)	atrament	atrament	Cf. MLW s.v. chalcanthum 1a and Frühneuhochdeutsches Wörterbuch s.v.
379	reubarbarum (rebarba)			Cf. 342a above.
380	reuponticum (reponticum)	wurzel von turkia		Ventura 405 calidum est et siccum. rapontikwurz in Grimm s.v. wahrhaft.
381	rafanus (rafani)	mer retich	meerrettich	Ventura 401 calidus est et siccus in tertio gradu.

74 Probably an error for crutzwúrtz, Daems 165, and 110a″ below.

Glossary 2

	Latin	German	Grimm	Notes
1″	amaracus, amariscus (armariacos)	*uncertain*		Daems 317; A8 amariscus (armariacum *F*), sansucus, maiorana, persa, olimbrum (elimbrion *A*) idem.
1a″	samsucus (sansucus)			
1b″	maiorana (maiarana)			
1c″	olimbrium (olibrium)			Daems 317*. Stirling s.v. olimblium, olimbrium. In spite of *Alphita*, there is good evidence for a form in -brium.
1d″	persa (persa)			Daems 317 and 649.
2″	adarasca (adarasca)			A225 adarasca id est elleborum albus.
2a″	elleborus albus (eleborum albus)	nise wurzin	nieswurz	Daems 191. Read perhaps ⟨wise⟩ nise wurzin.
3″	amantilla (amentila)	baldrion	baldrian	Daems 52. A9 amantilla potentilla marturella fu, ualeriana idem.
3a″		tiriaka	theriakskraut	Cf. Grimm s.v. wälsch (wälscher baldrian), but theriak itself is not attested for the plant.
3b″	potentilla (po⟨t⟩entila)			Cf. T24.
3c″	tormentilla (tormentila)			Cf. T24.
3d″	mantilla (mantila)			Distortion of amantilla?
3e″	phu (fu)			F67; Ventura 179.
3f″	ualeriana (ueleri⟨a⟩na)			
4″	alipiados (alimpiados)	sidelbast	seidelbast	A11 allippiados (alimpiados *F*) laureola herba catholica idem, cuius semen est coconidium.
4a″	coccus Cnidius (coconidion)			

(*cont.*)

	Latin	German	Grimm	Notes
5″	asphodelus (afodili)	wilde lok	wildlauch	Daems 508 (another plant is wildlauch, Grimm s.v., Marzell s.v.). A10 affodillus albucium centumcapita idem.
5a″	albucium (albucium)			
5b″	centumcapita (centumcapita)			
6″	agaricum (agaricum)	tanenswamin	tannenschwamm	Daems 48. A13 agaricus fungus abietis. Cf. 70 above.
7″	aristolochia rotunda (aristolongie rotunda)	hole wirze	hohlwurz	Daems 13. A18.
7a″		sinwol	sinwel	Grimm s.v. sinwel adj. 4) b) 'rund'. Here it may just be the adjective 'round', not a synonym of hohlwurz.
8″	anthemis (antimes)	kamileblumen	kamillenblume	Daems 112. A21 Anthemis camomilla idem.
8a″	camomilla[75] (camomila)			
9″	ami (ameos)	basiliensame	basiliensame	A31 ameos, nenuche, scintilla (ciminella *A*) idem. The identification with basiliensame is not found elsewhere; cf. MLW s.v. ami.
9a″	*uncertain*			
9b″	*uncertain*			
9c″	ciminella (cinimela)			C238 carui agreste ciminella piperidium ardeos (cf. MLW s.v.) idem. DMLBS s.v. cyminella.
10″	anemone (anemona)			A25 anemon papauer rubeum uel rufum; quando simpliciter ponitur, papauer album intelligitur.

75 In view of the close parallel in *Alphita* C223 camomilla anthemis idem, the best solution seems to be to emend קַפְּנֶלִין.

(*cont.*)

	Latin	German	Grimm	Notes
10a″	papauer rubeum (papaueris rubium)	rot magsam	roter magsam (mohnsamen)	Daems 361.
10b″	papauer album (papaueris albi)	wis magsam	weiszer mohnsamen	M42 miconium ... codium, papauer album.
10c″	codion[76] (codion)			
10d″	mecon (meco[77])			
11″	arnoglossa (arnoglosa)	spizwegerik	spitzwegerich	A50.
11a″		wissel or wiesel (?)		Marzell lists these words, but for other plants.
12″	adianthus (adiantus)	widertat	widertod	Daems 496 (widertodt). Marzell s.v. A55.
12a″	capillus Veneris (capili ueneris)			
13″	iris (iris)	schwertlin	schwertlein	Daems 235, Ventura 234; A59.
13a″		wisblumin	weiszblume	Other plants Marzell s.v. and Daems 112*.
13b″		lilien	lilie	
14″	ireos (ireos)			A59 yreos que habet album (sc. florem).
15″	acorus (acorus)			A59 acorus qui discernitur flore citrino.
15a″	gladiolus (gladiolus)			A59.

76 H. Frisk, *Griechisches etymologisches Wörterbuch*, has κώδεια as the headword, with κώδεα, κωδύα, κωδία as alternatives. The *Thesaurus linguae Latinae* s.v. codia, ae does not prefer one option, A. Souter, *A Glossary of Later Latin to 600 A.D.*, Oxford 1949, lists both *codia* and *codya*, probably without having reflected on the problem. J. André, *Lexique des termes de botanique en latin*, Paris 1956, has *codia, ae* and *codion, i* for the same plant (like MLW), but no entry whatsoever in his later work, *Les noms de plantes dans la Rome antique*, Paris 1985. I believe that *codion* originated from κωδειῶν, i.e., the gen. plur. of the word, found in the common preparation διὰ κωδειῶν. *codium* (as in M42) would then be an attempt at returning a perceived Greek nom. sing. n. to its correct Latin form.

77 The form *meco* (for regular *mecon* from Greek μήκων), gen. *meconis* is not attested but possible. But in view of *Alphita*, an emendation (*miconium*) seems attractive.

(*cont.*)

	Latin	German	Grimm	Notes
16″	alleluia (aleluia)	gukes luk	kuckuck-slauch	A67; Daems 61, Grimm s.v. kuckukslauch (sic!), Südhessisches Wörterbuch s.v.
17″	elaterium (elacterium[78])			E9 elacterium, succus cucumeris agrestis idem.
18″	*uncertain*			
18a″	*uncertain*			
19″	*herba Apollinis (erba apolonis)			herba Apollinis does not seem to be attested elsewhere, herba Apollinaris is different.
19a″		raden	raden	
20″	herba pedicularis (erba fiticularis)	wilde nelken	wildnelke	Not equivalent in Grimm s.v., cf. also Daems for other plants with that German name.
21″	intuba (intoba)	wege wise	wegeweise	I1 intiba (intuba *MDc*), solsequium, cicorea sponsaque solis idem, eliotropia, cuius flos est dionisia, eadem dicitur.
21a″	solsequium (solseqiom)			
21b″	dionysia (dionisia)			Cf. Grimm s.v. sonnenwirbel.
22″	hypocistis (ipoquistidos)	swamp	schwamm (= fungus)	I6 ipoquistidos est succus fungi qui nascitur ad pedem rose canine. Cf. Daems 268* tannenswamb.
22a″		hundsrosin	hundsrose	Literal translation of rosa canina.
23″	barba Iouis (barba iouis)			
23a″	stoechas (sticados citrinum)	wolgemut	wohlgemut	Daems 431, 88 and 720b. S13 sticados … citrinum idem est quod barba iouis; Ventura 429. Daems, Marzell and Grimm list other plants called 'wohlgemut'.

78 -ct- often represents simple t (or double t) in Romance areas at that time and is a hypercorrect spelling (like *micto* 'send' for *mitto*), because -ct- in Latin words developed into -t- or -tt-, e.g. factum → It. fatto. Cf. the spelling with an additional -c- not justified by the

(*cont.*)

	Latin	German	Grimm	Notes
23b″		*uncertain*		
23c″	testiculus uulpis	*uncertain*		See Daems 729* for another plant.
23d″		*uncertain*		
24″	bryonia (brironia)	wildkurbis	wildkürbis	B5. brironia is not attested so far.
25″	brathy (bracteos)	sevenbom	sevenbaum	B11. Cf. 139 and 258 above.
25a″	sabina (sauina)			
26″	buglossa (buglosa)	ohsenzung	ochsenzunge	B26.
27″	blitus (blitus)	ohsenougen	ochsenauge	B27 blitus ortus coxalidos[79] idem. Cf. Mensching 84,34. No explanation in García González. Many different plants in Marzell.
27a″	ortus (ortus)			Not in Stirling.
28″	bardana (bardana)			B28 bardana, lappa maior siue lappa inuersa idem.
28a″	lappa inuersa (lapa inuersa)			
28b″	maior (maior)	gros latik	groszlattich	Cf. Daems 520.
29″	bistorta (bistorta)			B30 bistorta herba est.
29a″	herba (erba)			
29b″	blita (blita)			
29c″		melde	melde	
30″	blita (blita)	mangolt	mangold	B33?
30a″		romeskol	römischer kohl	Daems 89.
31″	borago (borago)	borase	boretsch	Ventura 62. B40.
32″	bruncus[80] (bruncus)			B65 bruncus, cuscute, rasca lini idem.

etymology, 121, 139, and 188 above, and 77″ below. On the other hand, German lattich (168 above) < Lat. lactuca probably derives directly from latt-.

79 coxalis (or coxalidos, as a plant name) is not in DMLBS or Stirling; MLW s.v. coxalidas refers to caucalis, which fails to convince me.

80 Stirling s.v. *bruncus* wrongly quotes CGL 3,618,38 *bruncos id est guttor*, because *bruncos* = βρόγχος; cf. ThlL s.v. *guttur*.

(*cont.*)

	Latin	German	Grimm	Notes
32a″	cuscuta (cuscute)	side	seide	Cf. 37a.
33″	basilica (basilica)			B66 basilica, draguntea, serpentaria idem.
33a″	dracontea (draguntea)			
34″	bismalua (bismalva)	ibesch	eibisch	B63.
35″	cnicus (gnicus)	saferon in dem garten		G15 gnicus crocus ortensis. Daems 564. Cf. 179″.
36″	gramen (gramen)	wurzel von dem grasen	graswurzel	Other plants Grimm s.v. G54 gramen est nomen cuiuslibet herbe, tamen specialiter accipitur in medicina pro quadam herba cuius radix usualiter ponitur in oximelle …
37″	gruncus (gluncus[81])			G62 gruncus cuscute idem.
37a″	cuscuta (cuscuta)	side	seide	Cf. 32a.
38″	gariofilata (gariofilata)	benedicte	benedicte	Daems 248.
38a″	auancia (auancia)			S166 sanamunda, auancia idem.
38b″	sanamunda (sanamonda)			
39″	deronica (deronica)			D5 deronica siue ueronica, radix est parua …
39a″	ueronica (ueronica)			
40″	damnis (damnis)	*loreole?		Daems 629*. D7 dampnis laurus idem, inde dampnileon, id est oleum laurinum.
40a″	oleum laurinum (oleo laurinum)			
41″	dracunculus (dragunculus)	naterwurz	natterwurz	Daems 116.
41a″	dracontea (dragontea)			D9 draguntea, serpentaria, colubrina … idem.
42″	dendrolibanus (dendrolibanus)			D10 dendrolibanum … ros marinus idem; Ventura 408

81 *gluncus* is a dissimilation for *gruncus*.

(*cont.*)

	Latin	German	Grimm	Notes
42a″	anthos (antus)			A38 anthos flos roris marini.[82]
42b″	rosmarinus (rosmarinus)			
43″	dipparus (dipari)			Daems 369. Or read dipparis here.
43a″	polypodium (polipodion)	stenwurz	steinwurz	P6.
44″	dardana (dardana)	ros huf	roszhuf	Stirling s.v. dardana; Grimm and Marzell s.v.
45″	dens equinus (dens equinus)			D14 dens equinus sulfuraca.[83]
45a″	sulfurata (sulforata)			
46″	dactylus (dactili)			
47″	*uncertain*	hundsbis	hundsbisz	Marzell s.v.
48″	uirga pastoris (uirga pastoris)	wilde karten	wilde karde	Other plants in Marzell.
49″	uerrucaria (uerucaria)			V20 uerrucaria herba est.
50″	uerbena (uerbena)	iserharte	eisenhart	Daems 471. V41.
51″	zinziber (sinsiberis)	ingber	ingwer	Daems 486.
52″	zizania (sisania)	rate	raden	Daems 488.
52a″		zuker	zucker	Daems 487. It probably appears here because of an error in the compilation or transmission.
53″	zeduaria (situaria)			Daems 485. Z10 zedoarium radix est.
54″	tamariscus (tamariscus)			T4.
54a″		prume bom	prumebaum	This cannot be correct, because prume, praume, pfraume = pflaume (plum).
55″	tithymallus (titimalus)	wolfesmilk	wolfsmilch	T7 titimallus huius septem sunt species.

82 Add *Alphita* in MLW s.v. 1. *anthos.

83 For the variation between *sulfurac-* and *sulfurat-*, cf. Mensching p. 101 n. 14.

(*cont.*)

	Latin	German	Grimm	Notes
56″	turbith (turbit)			T12 turbith radix est.
57″	thapsia (tapsia)			T13 tapsia herba est que inflat uultum terentis[84] (tenentis *AVPQ*).
58″	tirus[85] (tirus)			T23 tirus est serpens.
59″	tormentilla (tormentila)			T24 tormentilla herba est.
60″	tartarum (tartarum)	winstain	weinstein	T2.
61″	genistula (jenistula)	primen	pfrimmen; pfriemen	Daems 594. G8 genestula genesta idem.
61a″	genista (jeniste)			
62″	elelisphacus (lilifagus)	wilde selbe	wilder salbei	L1 lilifagus saluia agrestis.
63″	lithospermon[86] (litospermatis)	stainbreksame	steinbrechsame	L2 litospermatis semen saxifrage.
64″	libanotis (libanotidos)	rosmarin[87] (rosmarine)	rosmarin	Daems 693. L108 libanothis id est flos roris marini.
65″	leporis priapiscus[88] (leporis priapiscos)			Daems 729*. L5 leporina priapiscus, herba satirion idem.
65a″	satyrion (satirion)			
66″	lauendula (lauendula)			L7 lauendula saluia agrestis idem.
66a″	saluia agrestis	wilde selbe	wilder salbei	

84 Cf. Haars 237, so it would make better sense to read *infla⟨mma⟩t uultum* (or *multum*) *tenentis*, "causes (severe) inflammation in the person holding (or touching) it."

85 θηρός is gen. sing. of θήρ nom. 'wild animal,' not necessarily a snake, cf. García González.

86 *litospermatis* must be a correction by somebody who knew that seed, in Greek, is σπέρμα (with the genitive σπέρματος), and not σπέρμον. The correct Greek name is λιθόσπερμον.

87 According to Grimm, the German word is only used from the 15th century onwards.

88 *leporis priapus* Daems 729*; *priapiscus* is the Greek diminutive. García González prints *priapismus*; and although this appears, e.g., in Matthaeus Silvaticus, it has no authority. Ventura 431 *priapiscus* (sic; *priapicus* in Ventura p. 722 and the index is an error). Cf. Mensching p. 123 n. 5 and Rufinus p. 281 *Synonima. Satyrion, id est, priapiscus uel testiculi leporis.*

(*cont.*)

	Latin	German	Grimm	Notes
67″	linozostis (linotides)	schis melde	scheiszmelde	Daems 315. L14 linozotis mercurialis linotides ... Cf. Marzell s.v. and Grimm s.v. scheiszkraut.
67a″	mercurialis (mercorialis)			
68″	linaria (linaria)			Daems 291. L6 linaria herba est similis esule, excepto quod lac non habet.
68a″	esula (esula)			
69″	lilium (lilium)			L12 lilium et ligustrum, quasi agreste lilium ... This attempt at an etymology for ligustrum is mistaken (in spite of Daems 278), lilium is not synonymous with ligustrum.
69a″	ligustrum (ligustrum)	wedewinde	wehdwinde	Grimm s.v. wehdwinde 3).
70″	lingua auis (linguam auis)	vogelzunge	vogelzunge	L15.
71″	lapathium acutum (lapacium acuti[!])	*uncertain* + spitzen		L19 lapacium ... due species, scilicet acutum et rotundum; Ventura 254.
71a″	*uncertain*			
72″	lapathium rotundum (lapacium rotunda[!])	roshufe	roszhuf	Cf. Grimm s.v. eselshuf.
73″	lithargyrum (litarjirum)	hefen von silber	hefe von silber	L22 litargirum fex est argenti.
74″	labrum Veneris (labrum ueneris)	wisdistel	weiszdistel	Daems 298. L30.
75″	lemnia (lemnias)			L26 lempnias auripigmentum idem, sed lempnia sfragidos terra est sigillata ...
75a″	auripigmentum (auripimentum)			Impossible to say how the two came to be confused.
76″	lacca (laca)			L28 lacca ... gumma est de qua et urina humana fit carminium.
76a″	gumma (guma)			

(*cont.*)

	Latin	German	Grimm	Notes
77″	lathyris (lactiridis)	sprinc wurz	springwurz	Daems 563. L38 lacterides id est catapucie, nomen est herbe et seminis eiusdem.
77a″	cataputia (catapucia)			
78″	lupulus (lupulus)	hoppe	hopfen	L54.
79″	laureola (laureola)	zidelbast	zeidelbast	Daems 169.
79a″		zigelinde	zilinde	Cf. Grimm s.v. ziegling.
80″	lineleon (lineleon)	linolei	(Diefenbach: linoley)	L74 lineleon id est oleum de semine lini.
81″	myrtus (mirtus)			M1 mirtus siue mirta idem, cuius semen est mirtillus, inde uinum et oleum mirtinum.
81a″	myrtilli (mirtilis)			
81b″	oleum myrtile (oleum mirtini[89])			Cf. Daems 638.
82″	marrubium (marubiom)	andorn	andorn	Daems 648. M18. Cf. 147″.
82a″	prasium (prasium)			
83″	macis (macis)	muskadenblumen	muskatenblume	M19.
84″	mabathematicon (mauabematicum)	kol	kohl	M28. Daems 344.
85″	millefolium (milefolium)	garwe	garbe	M32 millefolium minor ambrosia idem.
85a″	ambrosia minor (ambrosia mina[!])			
86″	marsilium (marsiliom)	nacht schade	nachtschatten	Daems 617. M40 marsilium, faba lupina idem.
86a″	faba lupina (faua lupina)			

89 ThlL s.v. corrects *oleum myrtile* (attested only once) in *myrtite*; in view of *Alphita*, it seems only possible to read *myrtinum* here.

(*cont.*)

	Latin	German	Grimm	Notes
87″	meconium (miconiom)	wis magsam	weiszer mohnsamen	Daems 361. M42 miconium hic comedio (cf. MLW s.v.).
87a″	*comida (comida[90])			'WoQ probably renders 'ok' (= also).
88″	magnes (mangnes)			
89″	mala siluestria (mala siluestria)	epel	äpfel	M49 mala maciana exponimus mala siluestria, sed uulgari Hyspanorum mala usualia, etiam domestica, dicuntur maciana.
89a″		zame un wilde holzepel	zahme und wilde holzäpfel	
90″	myrica (mirica)	heide	heide	Daems 319. M54 mirica genesta idem.
90a″	genista (jenista)	prame	brame	Daems 594.
91″	myotis (miotis)			M55 miotis herba est nobis ignota.
92″	mespila (mespila)	mispeln	mispeln	M62.
93″	muscus (muscus)	bisem	bisam	M64. Cf. Grimm s.v. bisam for bisem.
94″	musa (musa)			M66 musa fructus est in quo dicunt primum parentem peccasse ...
95″	micinum (micinum)			M117 micinum id est reuocatiuum.
95a″	minium[91] (minium)			M68 minium color est pictorum et scriptorum.
96″	musceleon (musceleon)	bisam	bisam	M69.
97″	molybdaenum (molipdenum)	bli	blei	M85 molipdinum id est plumb[e]um.[92]
98″	murion (mirion)			Daems 380. M76 murion id est auricula muris.

90 Different is Mensching 100,28 Comide (Comida M), i. goma arauiga (= gummi Arabicum).

91 Certainly not German; the mixup must be due to a problem (corruption) in the Ms that was copied.

92 In our opinion, García González is mistaken in preferring *plumbeum* and deriving *molipdinum* from μολύβδινον, which is indeed an adjective.

(*cont.*)

	Latin	German	Grimm	Notes
98a″	auricula muris (auricla moris)	musor	mausohr	
99″	nymphaea (ninfea)			N20 nimphea est herba crescens in aquis.
100″	narca (narcos[93])	... macht slafen	... macht schlafen	N24 narca piscis est ... inde narcoticum, omne medicamen stuporiferum.
101″	naphtha (napta)			N28 napta id est petroleum rubei coloris.
101a″	petroleum (pitirolion)	un ist rote⟨r⟩ varwe	und ist roter farbe	
102″	nucleus (nucleus)	pinien korner	pinienkörner	N30 nucleus quando simpliciter ponitur, de nucleo pinee[94] intelligitur. Cf. 116.
103″	nileos[95] (nileos)	semde	semde	Daems 272*. N14 nileos iuncus est cuius radix assimilatur galange.
103a″		*uncertain* + galgan	galgan	The German word preceding galgan could be wilt (cf. Grimm s.v. galgan, Daems 114).
104″	sagapenum (sagapinum)			S1 sagapinum siue serapinum, gumma est.
104a″	serapinum (serapinum)			
105″	seseli (sesilium[96])			S2 siseleos siler montanum idem.

93 *narcos* is found in some mss. of the *Alphita*, cf. further N25 in Mensching.

94 DMLBS defines *pinea* as 'pine cone', which fits Daems 367; might it also mean 'pine tree' (classical Latin *pinus*, from which the adjective *pineus, a, um* is derived)?

95 Not in DMLBS or Stirling; *nilion* in Stirling (*Ranunculus sceleratus* L.) is different. The easiest explanation seems to be to read it as Νειλαῖος, adjective of Νεῖλος 'Nile', i.e., (rush) from the Nile.

96 *siseleum* in André s.v. *seselis*, a form that is also in some Mss of the *Alphita* and in Marcell. *med.* 20.88 and 20.101 (both recipes without an identified source); CGL 3.273,67; see Winkler, app. crit., in *Plin. phys. Flor.-Prag.* 1.58.25. (σέσελι, gen. σεσέλεως → *seseleos* → *seseleum* → *seselei*)

(*cont.*)

	Latin	German	Grimm	Notes
105a″	siler montanum (sileris montanis)			sileris montanis is attested (as is the correct sileris montani) in Mensching, cf. the index there and cf. 154a.
106″	squinantum (squinantum)	stro	stroh	Daems 445. S7 squinantum palea camelorum.[97]
107″	stoechas (sticados)	geln blumen		Daems 431 and 720. S13 sticados huius due sunt species, scilicet citrinum et arabicum. Other plants in Marzell s.v. gelbblume.
107a″		wolgemut	wohlgemut	Other plants in Marzell.
108″	satyrion (satirion)			S16 satirion herba est cuius radix competit multum medicine.
109″	scabiosa (s⟨c⟩abiosa)			S35.
110″	senecio (senec⟨i⟩on)			Daems 422 attests the form in -on, as does DMLBS. S36 senecio cardus benedictus idem.
110a″	cardus benedictus	kruzwurz	kreuzwurz	Daems 165. Cf. 368.
111″	senacio (senacio)	brunenkrese	brunnenkresse	S36 … sed senacio est nasturcium aquaticum quod alio nomine dicitur cresso, cressonis.
112″	sandalum (sandali)	rot wis gel	rot weisz gelb	S56 sandalus, huius tres sunt species, scilicet albus, rubeus et citrinus.
113″	serpyllum (serpelum)			S60 serpillum herpillum idem.
113a″	herpyllum (harpilom)	?? in der erden[98]	… in der erde	
114″	centaurea (sentaurea)			C45.
115″	sperma (sperma)			S71 sperma interpretatur semen.

97 kamelstroh Grimm s.v. kamelheu.

98 Ventura 460 *super terram serpit.*

(*cont.*)

	Latin	German	Grimm	Notes
116″	strobilus (strobili[99])	pinien korner	pinienkörner	S81. Cf. 102 above.
117″	sycomorus (sicomorus)			S83 sicomorus id est ficus fatua, arbor est cuius fructus dicuntur siccamina.
117a″	ficus fatua (ficus fatua)			
117b″	sycamina (sicamina)			
118″	scorpio (*scorpia)			S86 scorpio animal est uenenosum.
119″	sigillum sancte Marie (sigilum sante merie)			Daems 706. S93 sigillum sancte Marie herba est.
120″	smirnis[100] (smirnis)			S116 smirnis betonica idem. Cf. Mensching 149,6 and n. 114 and 282 above.
120a″	betonica (betonica)	betonia	betonie	
121″	sister (sister)			S119 sister anetum agreste.
121a″	anethum agreste	wilde til	wilder dill	Daems 314.
122″	selinum (selinum)	epe sam	eppichsamen	S121 selinum id est semen apii.
123″	sichen (siken)	wilde eberzen	wilder eberzahn[101]	A65 abrotanum … sed sichen armenicum est abrotanum agreste.
124″	scariola (scariola)			Daems 202, 450 and 572. S205 scariola endiuia.
124a″	endiuia (endiuia)	su distel	saudistel	
125″	saponaria (saponaria)	raden	raden	Cannot be the same as B48, if the German is correct.

99 The form *strobile* (first declension plural) in *Alphita* seems possible, analogous with *pinee* (sc. *nuces*).

100 The form of the word is not stable and well attested; DMLBS and Stirling do not help. García González, it seems, has not recognised the problem.

101 Marzell only has eberwurz for *Artemisia abrotanum* L. (eberzahn in Grimm is different; eberwurz in Daems is also used for other plants.) *sichen* is not in DMLBS or Stirling. Mensching p. 64 n. 100 has *sychen armenicum*, the same spelling as García González's Ms *U*.

(*cont.*)

	Latin	German	Grimm	Notes
126″	sulphurata (sulfurata)			S39 (and D14) sulphuraca and sulfuraca,[102] cf. Daems 313 and 260*.
127″	filipendula (filipendula)			F1. Daems 216 cites *Alphita* 66[103] (also quoted in DMLBS): filipendula … habet multos testiculos in radice.
128″	finicea[104] (finicea)	daitel	*uncertain*	Cf. Daems 189 finitia and 153 above.
129″	pilosa (pilosa)	bapel	pappel	Daems 308*. Probably Grimm s.v. pappel (= malve).[105]
129a″	Syriacus (ciriacus)			Daems 222 (pappelen blům). F4 flos siriacus (cf. Stirling s.v.), flos malue idem.
130″	feniculata (feniculata)			Daems 364. F9 feniculata herba est longa et gracilis que nascitur in aquis.[106]
131″	fenum Graecum (fenigreca)		(feine grete)	Daems 210. Grimm s.v. grete 3) d).
132″	flos malue? (*uncertain*)			F4; identification uncertain.[107] Cf. 129a above and Mensching 110,4 Flos siriacus, id est flor de malua.
133″	folium (folium)	bleder von nelkin	blätter von nelken	F25 folium quando simpliciter ponitur, pro foliis gariofilorum intelligitur.

102 There is no point in distinguishing *sulphuraca* and *sulfuraca*, purely graphic variants. The correct Latin form, in any case, is the one we find here, i.e., *sulfurata*, also (as *sulphurata*) transmitted by Mss *FA* of the *Alphita*.

103 Mowat's edition, not in García González. The Hebrew suggests that the words were part of at least some Mss of *Alphita*.

104 Stirling s.v. finitia and phoenicea seem close, but preferable seems to be F5 finicon (finitio *D* finicio *F*) dactilus palme …, with daitel (or detel) as an unattested form of dattel.

105 Stirling lists other species s.v. pilosa and pilosella.

106 García González identifies *feniculata*, probably correctly, with *Peucedanum officinale* L., which fits *longa et gracilis*; *in aquis* would then mean 'in waterlogged environments'. This seems preferable to Stirling s.v. feniculum aquaticum and feniculum aquaticum galericulatum = *Callitriche cophocarpa* Sendtner (Stirling and DMLBS have no entry *feniculata*).

107 The flowers of mallows are not yellow.

(*cont.*)

	Latin	German	Grimm	Notes
134″	flaura (flaura)			Daems 209. F7; some mss. add herba ualde amara, unde optime necat uermes interius et exterius.[108] Cf. Stirling s.v.
135″	faua (faba)			F32 faba est quedam herba.
136″	flictena (flictina)			F36 flectena bulla (bulba *A*) idem.
136a″	bulba[109] (bolba)			
137″	fel terre (fel tere)	tusint gildin	tausendgül-denkraut	F61 fel terre, centaurea idem.
138″	filix quercina (filicis quercina)			Daems 217. F72 filex[110] quercina, polipodium idem.
138a″	polypodium (polipo-dio)			
139″	ferrugo (ferrogo)			F73.
139a″	ferrarium (ferarium)	das man findit im leschtrog	das man im löschtrog findet	F74 ferrarium est quod inuenitur in trunco[111] in quo faber refrigerat forcipes, unde ipsa aqua ferraria dicitur.
140″	peucedanum (pau-cedanus)			Daems 364. P2 peucedanum fe-niculus porcinus.
140a″	feniculus porcinus (weniculus[112] por-cinus)			Cf. Grimm s.v. saufenchel.
141″	parietaria[113] (pali-taria)	nacht un tak	nacht und tag	P9. Marzell s.v. tag und nacht. Daems 366. Cf. 145.

108 A very bitter plant, and for this reason it kills worms inside and outside.
109 בּוּלְבָא must be a mistake for בולא *bulla* (MLW).
110 For variant spellings, cf. ThlL s.v. filix.
111 This meaning is recorded in DMLBS s.v. truncus 5b.
112 An instance where WW represents /f/.
113 Because of the German translation, reading *pulicaria* seems less likely, especially since *pulicaria* occurs immediately after the following entry at 142a″.

(*cont.*)

	Latin	German	Grimm	Notes
142″	psyllium (psiliom)			P4 Psillium herba est, policaris dicitur.
142a″	pulicaria (policaria)			P3 pollicaria.
142b″	palma Christi (palma cristi)			P126;[114] cf. Stirling s.v.
143″	priapus (priapus)	menschen zakel	menschenzagel[115]	P126 palma Christi priapus idem;[116] cf. P10 pentadactilus … palma Christi … priapus idem.
144″	pentadactylus (pentodactilis)			P10 pentadactilus, custos ortorum.[117]
144a″	custos (custos)			
145″	parietaria (paritaria)			P9 paritaria perdiciados. Cf. 141.
145a″	perdicias (paricidiados[118])			
146″	puleium regale (puleum regale)	polai	polei	P12 pulegium regale est gliconium, et est aliud pulegium ceruinum.
146a″	glyconium[119] (gliconiom)			
146b″	puleium ceruinum (pulei ceruinum)			
147″	prasium (prasium)	andorn	andorn	P20 prassium[120] est marrubium album. Cf. 82.

114 This suggests a mistake in the order of entries; a new entry should obviously start with *palma Christi*.

115 zagel (tail) is first used of animals, cf. Grimm s.v.

116 No blasphemy intended.

117 The protector of gardens is Priapus (e.g. Priap. 1.5 *hortorum custos*).

118 For variants (but not the one in this glossary), see Mensching p. 373.

119 Obviously a well-meant but incorrect form for Greek γλήχων based on plant names with *glycy-* 'sweet'.

120 We fail to understand why García González chooses *prassum* instead of *prassium* (mss. *HBFA*), πράσιον, and *prassium* occurring immediately after; cf. also Mensching p. 376, where -i- is attested a number of times. But cf. DMLBS s.v. prason.

(*cont.*)

	Latin	German	Grimm	Notes
147a″	marrubium album (marobium album)			
148″	peniculus (penicolus)			P25 penicellus (peniculus *F*) spongia idem.[121]
148a″	spongia (sponjia)	merschwamp	meerschwamm	
149″	polygonia (poligonii)	wegetrete	wegetritt	Daems 166. P23 poligonia poligonium.
149a″	polygonium (poligoniom)			
150″	peristereon orthon (peristereon orton)	iserharte	eisenhart	Daems 471. P26 peristereon orton uerbena recta. Stirling s.v.
150a″	uerbena recta (uerbena recta)			
151″	pentaphyllon (pentafilon)	funf finger[122]	fünffinger	Daems 668. P27.
152″	propoleos (propolion)	wiswachs	weiszwachs	Daems 387. P28 propoleos est cera alba.
153″	pipinella (pipinela)	bibinele	pimpernell	Daems 372. P29 pimpinella herba est multum similis saxifrage.
153a″	saxifraga (saxifraga)			
154″	plato⟨cyminum⟩ (plata)			P32 platociminum id est siler montanum; cf. Grimm s.v. siler.
154a″	siler montanum (sileris montanis)			Cf. 105a above.
155″	picus?[123]	wis + *uncertain*	weisz + *uncertain*	

121 Cf. ThlL s.v. (made from hairs or a sponge).

122 See Grimm s.v. fünfblatt and Marzell s.v. fünffingerkraut for plants with that name.

123 *picus* 'woodpecker'; if read *ficus*, it would mean fig or fig tree, which has a bark that may be described as grey and justify 'wis bo⟨r⟩ke' as a German rendering.

(*cont.*)

	Latin	German	Grimm	Notes
156″	sidia (psidia[124])	slote von granat epel	schlote[125] von granat-äpfeln	P41 psidia est cortex mali granati.
157″	peplum[126] (peplom)	*uncertain* + distel	*uncertain* + distel	P48 peplum ... quoddam genus cardui in cuius summitate nascuntur quasi fila subtilissima ...
158″	pellicinum (pelicinom)			P53 pellicinum herba est nobis ignota.
159″	perdicias (perdiciados)	sis melde	süsze melde[127]	Well attested, but not identifiable with certainty.
160″	cynoglossa (cinoglosa)	hunszunge	hundszunge	C65 cinoglossa lingua canis idem.
161″	chelidonia agrestis (celidonia agrestis)	wilde schelwurz	wilde schöllwurz	Daems 115. C56 celidonia agrestis.
162″	cymbalaria (cimbalaria)			Daems 147. C80 cimbalaria, cotilidon, umbilicus Veneris idem.
162a″	umbilicus (ombilicus)			
163″	cyclamen (ciclamen)	erdnus	erdnusz	Daems 151. C7 ciclamen ... malum terre idem.
164″	condisi (condisi)	slote von wiser niswirze	schlote der weiszen nieswurz	C24 condisi est cortex ellebori albi.
165″	cissos (kison)	ebich	epheu	Daems 200. C39 cisson id est edera. Cf. 182b″ below.
165a″	hedera (edera)			
166″	cocconidium (coconidion)	sidelbast	seidelbast	C40.

124 The form with p- is hypercorrect; σίδια is the plural of σίδιον, cf. García González. It does not occur in the old Latin translation (referred to as Dioscorides Longobardus) at Diosc. *mat. med.* 1.110.3.

125 The same word for *cortex* in 164 below, so probably not an error for 'schote'.

126 See DMLBS s.v. peplus 5. Cf. also Stirling s.v. peplos and peplum.

127 Marzell only has solte (= salty) melde.

(*cont.*)

	Latin	German	Grimm	Notes
167″	caniculata (caniculata)			C41 caniculata iusquiamus.
167a″	canicularis (canicolaris)			
167b″	iusquiamus (iusquiami)	bilsensamen	bilsensame	
168″	calamus aromaticus (calamus aromaticus)			C51.
169″	crassula (crasula)	stainpeper	steinpfeffer	C60.
170″	carpobalsamum (carpobalsam')			C62 carpobalsamum dicitur fructus balsami …
171″	cordumeni (cordumeni)	matkumel	mattenkümmel	C64 cordumeni carui agrestis idem. Cf. 183″.
171a″	caruum agreste (carui agreste)			Daems 157. C238 carui agreste. Cf. 183″.
172″	coronopodium (coronopodion)			Mensching 95,11 cornopodion, id est pes çeruino (and comm. ibid. p. 275). C69 cornopodium pes coruinus idem, herba est.
172a″	pes ceruinus[128] (pes ceruinos)	hirsfus	*hirschfusz	
173″	chrysomela (crisolima)			C73 Cochima, antipersica, crisomila idem, quod interpretatur mala aurea uulgari Prouincialium amoriaca. Cf. Mensching 94,17 and n. 98.
173a″	Provence (provinza)			
174″	carioca (carioca)	wilde morchen	wilde möhre	C82 carioca pastinaca agrestis idem. Daems 360.
174a″	pastinaca (pastinaca)			

128 The German translation makes it clear that the translator read *ceruinus*, not *coruinus*. Cf. Marzell s.v. rabenfuß; hirschfusz as a plant name is not attested.

(*cont.*)

	Latin	German	Grimm	Notes
175″	carambia (carambia)	*uncertain*		Cf. C89 cantabia (carambia *RBF* carabia *W*) genus caulis albi. (Mensching 95,4)
175a″		wiskol	weiszkohl	
176″	calamintha (calaminta)	stainminze	steinminze	C90.
177″	chamaeleon (cameleonta)			C101 cameleonta ... herba est de cuius flore fit coagulum.[129]
178″	crispula (crispula)			C129.
178a″	centumgrana (centom grana)	hundert korner	hundertkörner[130]	Daems 146. C130.
179″	crocus orientalis (crocus orientalis)	safron	safran	Cf. G15 gnicus crocus ortensis idem, et est alius orientalis qui dicitur safran. Cf. 35″ above.
180″	crocus hortensis (crocus ortencis)	wilde safron	wilder safran	
181″	conium (conium)			
181a″	cicuta (cicuta)	scherlink	schierling	C8 cicuta ... conium idem.
182″	carpocissus (carpocisi)			C230 carpocissi fructus edere idem.
182a″	fructus hedere (fructus edere)			
182b″		ebich	epheu	Cf. 165″ above.
183″	caruum agreste (caroe agreste)	wilde matkumel	wilder mattkümmel	C238 carui agreste. Cf. 171″ above and Mensching 76,26 and 96,6.
184″	custos hortorum (custos ortorom)	graslatek	*graslattich	
185″	colocynthis (coloquintide)			C6 colloquintida gelena, cucurbita Alexandrina idem. Mensching 91,9.
185a″	cucurbita Alexandrina (cocorbita alexandrina)			

129 The Hebrew translation "fatty substance" is not correct, cf. also Mensching 95,31.

130 Not in Marzell or Grimm.

(*cont.*)

	Latin	German	Grimm	Notes
186″	codium (codiom)	schwarze magen?	schwarzer mohn	Cf. M42 miconium ... codium, papauer album(!) idem.
187″	rodon[131] (rodon)	rose	rose	R1 rosa ... Item rodon, rosa idem ...
188″	rodostagma (rodostoma)	rosenwaser	rosenwasser	R1 rosa ... rodostoma, id est aqua rosata. DMLBS s.v. rhodostagma.
188a″	oxyrodon (oxirodon)	esig un rosen gemischt	essig und rosen[132] gemischt	R1 oxirodon, id est acetum mixtum cum oleo rosato.
189″	reu (reu)			
189a″	reubarbarum (reubarbar)			R9.
190″	rhus Syriacus (ros siriacos)	bapeleblumen	pappelblume[133]	R13. Daems 222.
191″	resta bouis (resta bouis)			R9.
192″	rumex (romex)			R25 rumex, huius sunt duo genera, scilicet ferens mora et sterilis.
193″	resina (resina)			R35 resina potest uocari omnis gumma. Item appropriatum est hoc uocabulum ad designandum gummam abietis, quando simpliciter inuenitur.
193a″		tane	tanne	

131 ῥόδων, gen. pl. of ῥόδον 'rose' (more likely than nom. or acc. sing.).

132 The German translation does not make clear that rose = oleum rosatum, a meaning not recorded in Grimm. Grimm s.v. rosenöl does not say that in medieval pharmacy, oleum rosatum etc. is not (as today) the oil pressed from rose petals but a preparation where rose petals are macerated or even boiled in oil, cf. Ventura 400, p. 684 Oleum rosarum sic fit etc.

133 In Daems, Marzell, and Grimm used for other plants because of the confusion of *rus* (*ros*) *Syriacus* and *flos Syriacus*.

Index of Terms in Hebrew Characters

Entries in Glossary 2 are marked with ″.

Index of Latin Terms

Usually, the form of the Latin nominative singular is given, unless the plural is current, e.g. *amygdala* (the form itself may also be nom. sing. f., cf. MLW). References to unrecognizable word forms, marked as "uncertain" in the lists, are omitted here.

Entries in Glossary 2 are marked with ″.

dendrolibanus 42″
dens equinus 45″
deronica 39
diagridium 154
dionysia 21b″
dipparus 43″
dracontea 33a″, 41a″
dracunculus 41″

ebulus 13, 68, 97
edera → hedera
elaterium 17
elelisphacus 189, 62″
elleborus → helleborus
ematites → lapis haematites
emblici 2 → myrobalani
emula → inula
endiuia 3, 124a″
entiana → gentiana
enula → inula
epatica → hepatica
epithymum 5a, 77
eruca 12, 74
erucula 12a
es ustum 8
esula 99, 68a″, e. maior 10, e. minor 10
eupatorium 1, 110
euphorbium 6, 29

faba lupina 86a″
faua 135″
fel terre 137″
feniculata 130″
feniculum 292
feniculus porcinus 140a″
fenum Graecum 265, 131″
ferrarium 139a″
ferrugo 139″
ficus fatua 117a″
filipendula 156a, 127″
filix quercina 138″
finicea 128″
flammula 308
flaura 134″
flictena 136″
flos malue 132″
folium (as a plant-name = folium caryophyllorum) 285, 133″
folium citrinum 295
fu → phu
fumitaria → fumitera
fumitera 306
fumus terre 305

galanga 144
galbanum 145
gallia muscata? 147
gariofilata 38
gelena 149
genista 61a″, 90a″
genistula 61
gentiana 14, 163
gerontea 150
gingiber → zingiber
git 148, 164
gladiolus 15a″
glutinum 271a
glyconium 146a″
glycyrrhiza → liquiricia
gnicus → cnicus
gramen 36
granum paradisi 146
gruncus 37
gumma 20a, 76a″

hedera 81, 94, 165a″, fructus hedere 182a″
helleborus 9, 46, h. albus 2a″
hepatica 7, 52, 76
herba + *uncertain* 59
herba Apollinis 19
herba pedicularis 20
herba perforata 44
hermodactylus 15, 50
herpyllum 113a″
hordeum 23
hyoscyamus 162, 167b″
hypericum 48
hypocistis 58, 22″
hyssopus → ysopus

Indus → myrobalani
intuba 21
inula 4, 11
inula campana 98
ireos → iris
iris 17, 51, 62, 95, 13″, 14″
iua 91
iuniperus 18, 166
iusquiamus → hyoscyamus

Index of German Terms

Entries in Glossary 2 are marked with ″.

Facsimiles

Collective volume with texts in Hebrew and German: *Shemot ha-Asavim*; and other texts; Ms Leiden, Universiteitsbibliotheek, Cod. Or. 4732/1 (SCAL 15), fols. 1a–17b

 | DOI:10.1163/9789004459380_008

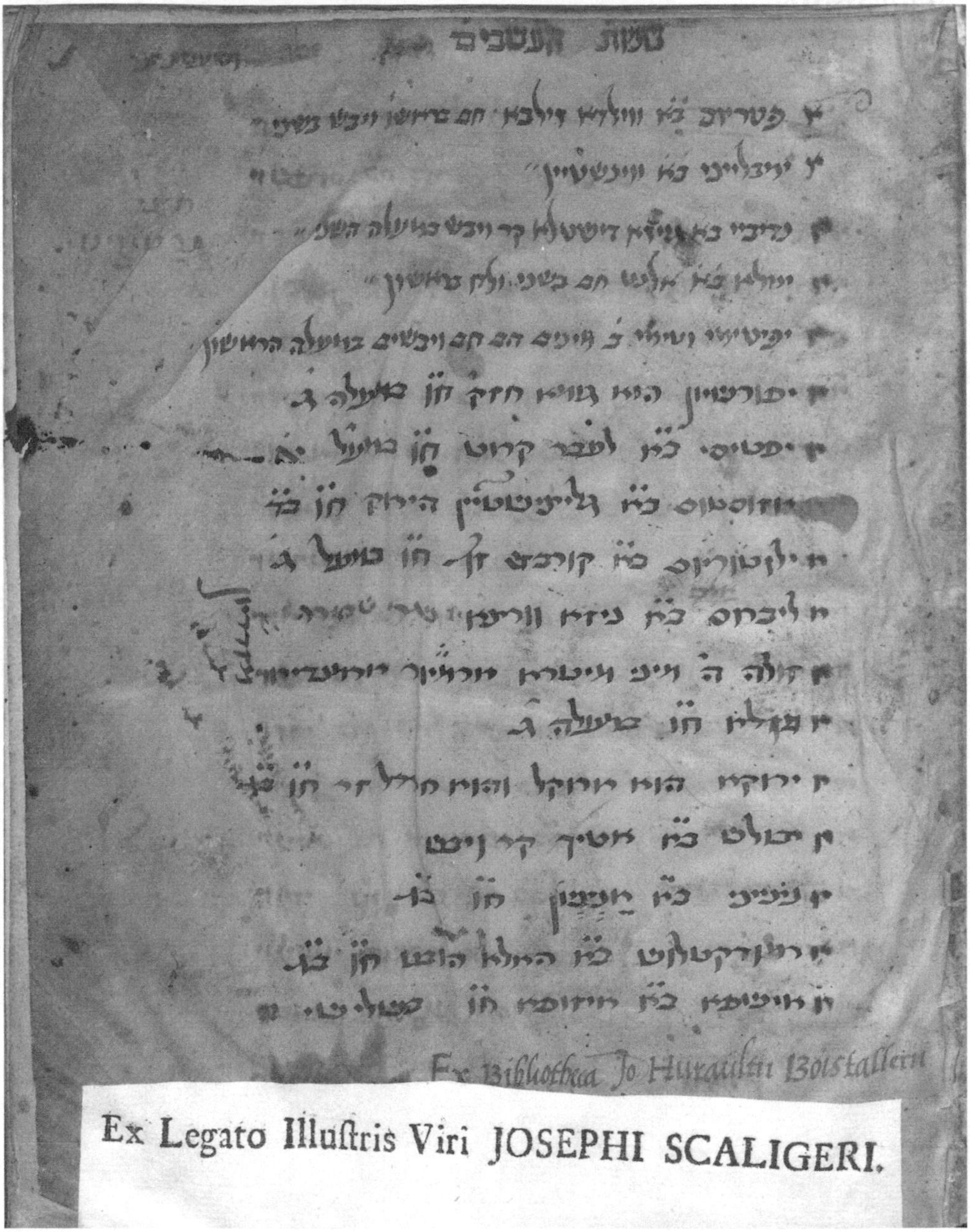
Ex Bibliotheca Jo Huraulti Boistallerii
Ex Legato Illustris Viri JOSEPHI SCALIGERI.

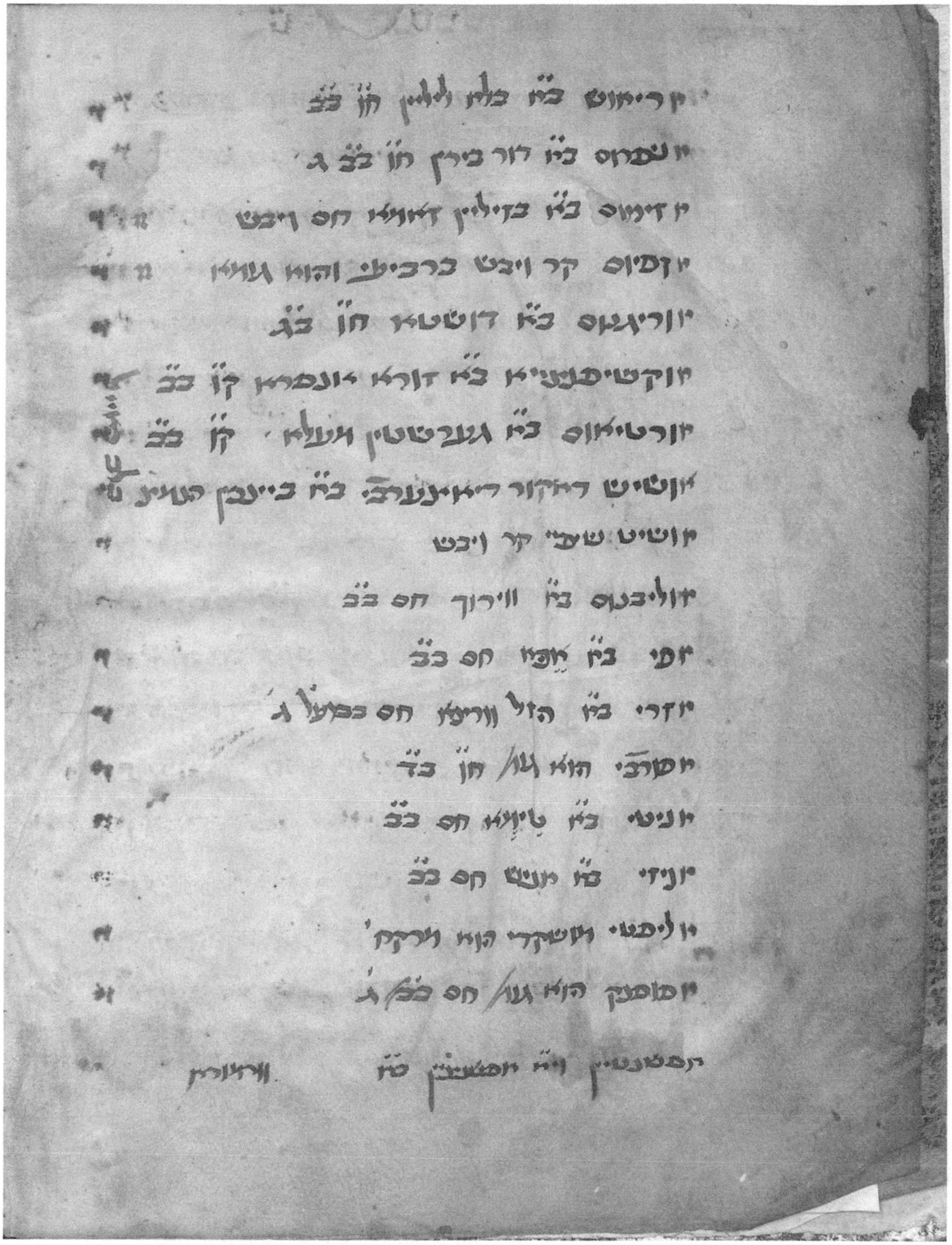

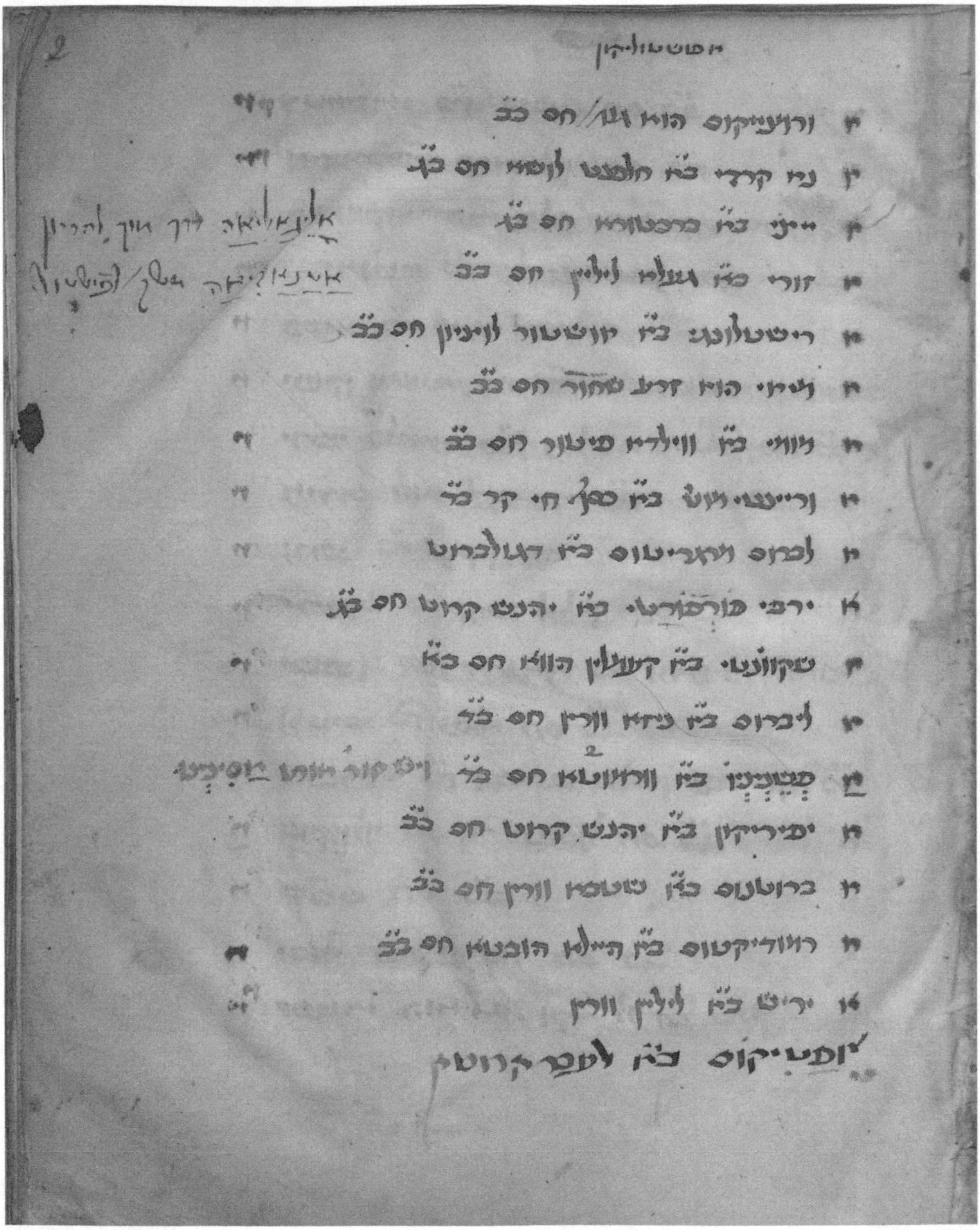
מפטטוליקין
ורונייקוס הוא גגו/ חם בב״
נוי קרדי ב״ה חלפטא לנשוא חם ב״ג
ייני ב״ה מרפטורא חם ב״ג
זורי ב״ה גגלא לולין חם ב״ב
רישטולוגי ב״ה יוסטור לוניין חם ב״ב
ליני הוא זרע שחור חם ב״ב
מווי ב״ה ווילדא פיטור חם ב״ב
ורייטני ב״ה סגן חי קר ב״ד
לפרס ומאריטוס ב״ה דגולברט
ירבי פורפורטי ב״ה יהנט קרוט חם ב״ג
שקוונטי ב״ה קעעלין הוואי חם ב״א
ליברוס ב״ה נידא וורן חם ב״ד
פטפני ב״ה ורווטא חם ב״ד
יפיריקון ב״ה יהנש קרוט חם ב״ב
ברוטנוס ב״ה שוטמא וורן חם ב״ב
רוודיקטוס ב״ה היילא הובטא חם ב״ב
ירינט ב״ה לולין וורן
יופטיקוס ב״ה לעבר קרוטף

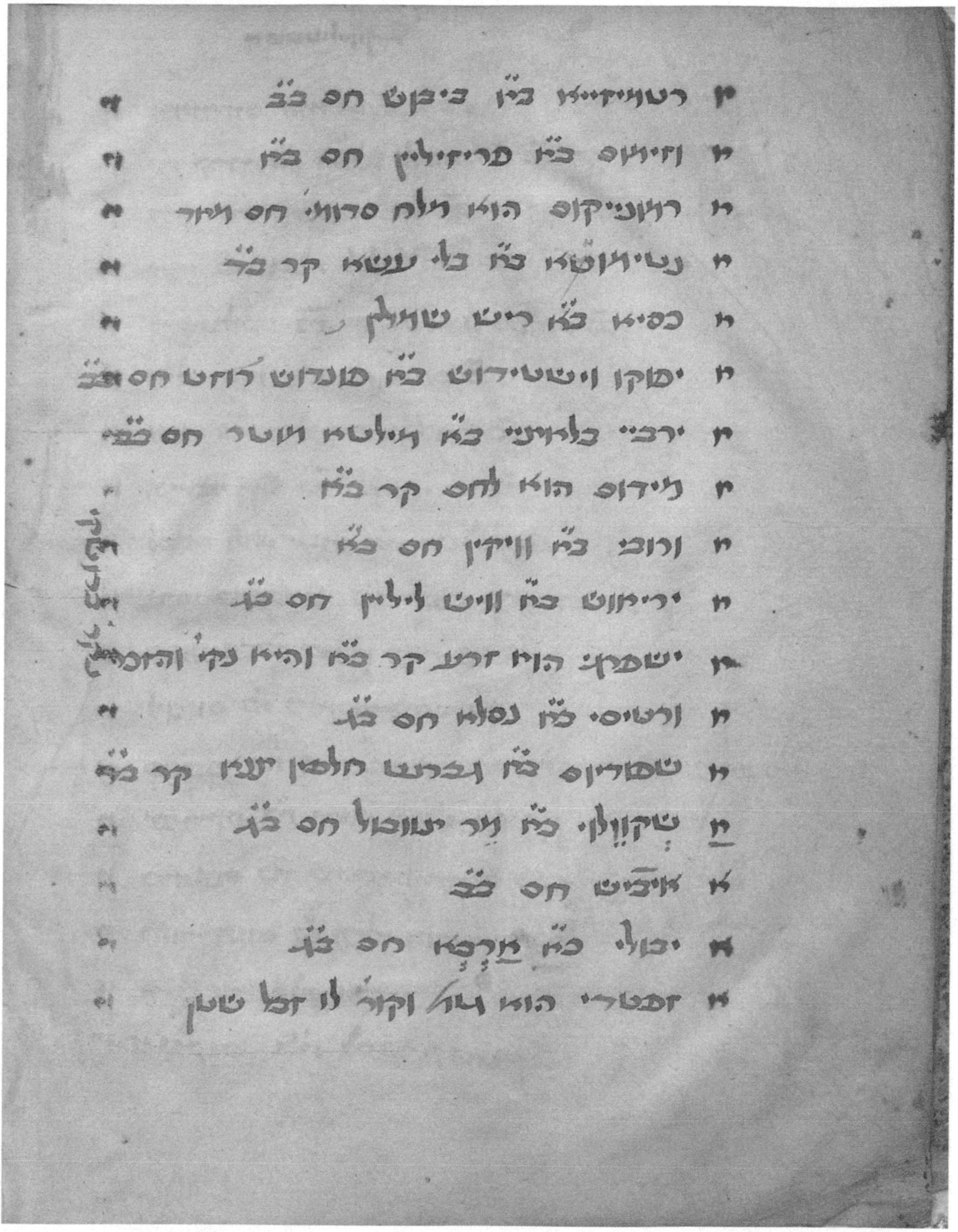
רטאמיידייאו ב״ן ביבנש חס ב״ב
וזיזופ ב״א פריזילין חס ב״ן
רמוניקופ הוא מלח סרומי חס מאד
נטירונשא ב״א בלי עשא קר ב״ד
כסיא ב״א ריש שמלך
יסקו וישטירוש ב״א מנדוש רוזט חס ב״ב
ירבי בלאנקי ב״א מילשא מוטר חס ב״ב
מידופ הוא לחס קר ב״ה
ורובי ב״א ווידין חס ב״א
ירימנש ב״א וויש זילין חס ב״ג
ישפקי הוא זרע קר ב״א והוא נקי והזמוק
ורטיסי מ״ן נסלא חס ב״ג
שפוריופ מ״ן גברטא חלמן יעני קר ב״ה
שקוולוי מ״ן מר יעונמל חס ב״ג
אויבוש חס ב״ב
יבולי מ״ן מרבא חס ב״ג
זפטרי הוא מור וקור לו זמל שטן

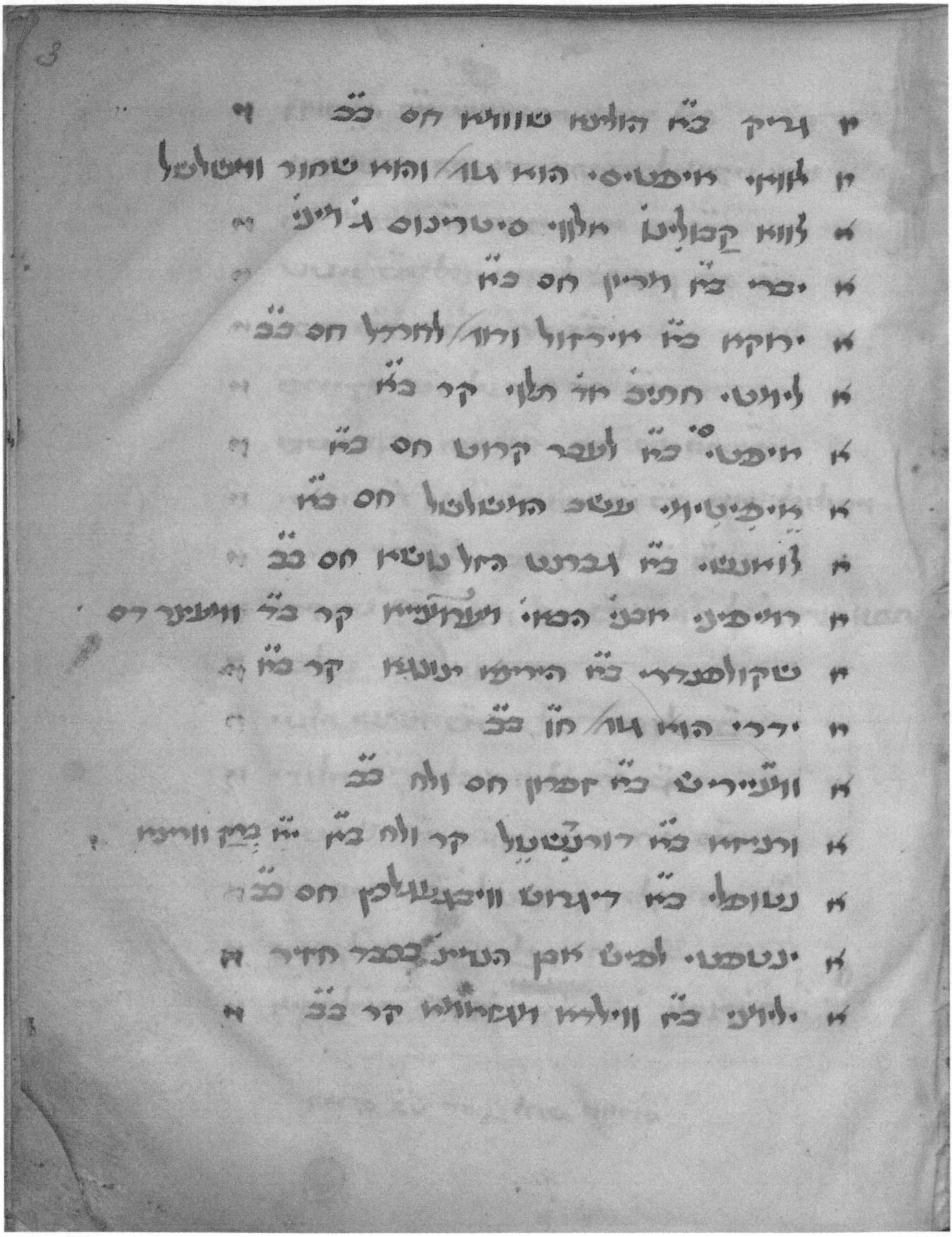

3

יו גריק בל״א הולנא שוורצא חם בב״

יו לאורי אימפטיסי הוא גוד/ והוא שחור ואשולטשל

א לווא קבוליטו אלווי סיטרינוס ג׳ריני

א יפרי בל״א מרין חם בא״

א ירוקא בל״א אירדול ורוד/ לחרדל חם בב״

א ליאטי חתיכ יוד׳ חלוי קר בא״

א אימפטי׳ בל״א לעבר קרוט חם בא״

א איפיטיאי עשב האישולטול חם בא״

א לואנשי בל״א גברטא הול טשא חם בב״

א רואפיני אכני המאי מערמיין קר בד״ וואנר דס

א שקולפנדרי בל״א הירשא ינונגא קר בא״

א ידרי הוא גוד/ חם בב״

א ואנייריט בל״א זמרון חם ולח בב״

א ורניזא בל״א דורנשטעל קר ולח בא״ ורנזא

א נעופלי בל״א ריגרוט וויבגשולכן חם בב״

א ינטשי לפיט אמן העירינ במבר חדיר

א ילוני בל״א ווילדא מגשולא קר בב״

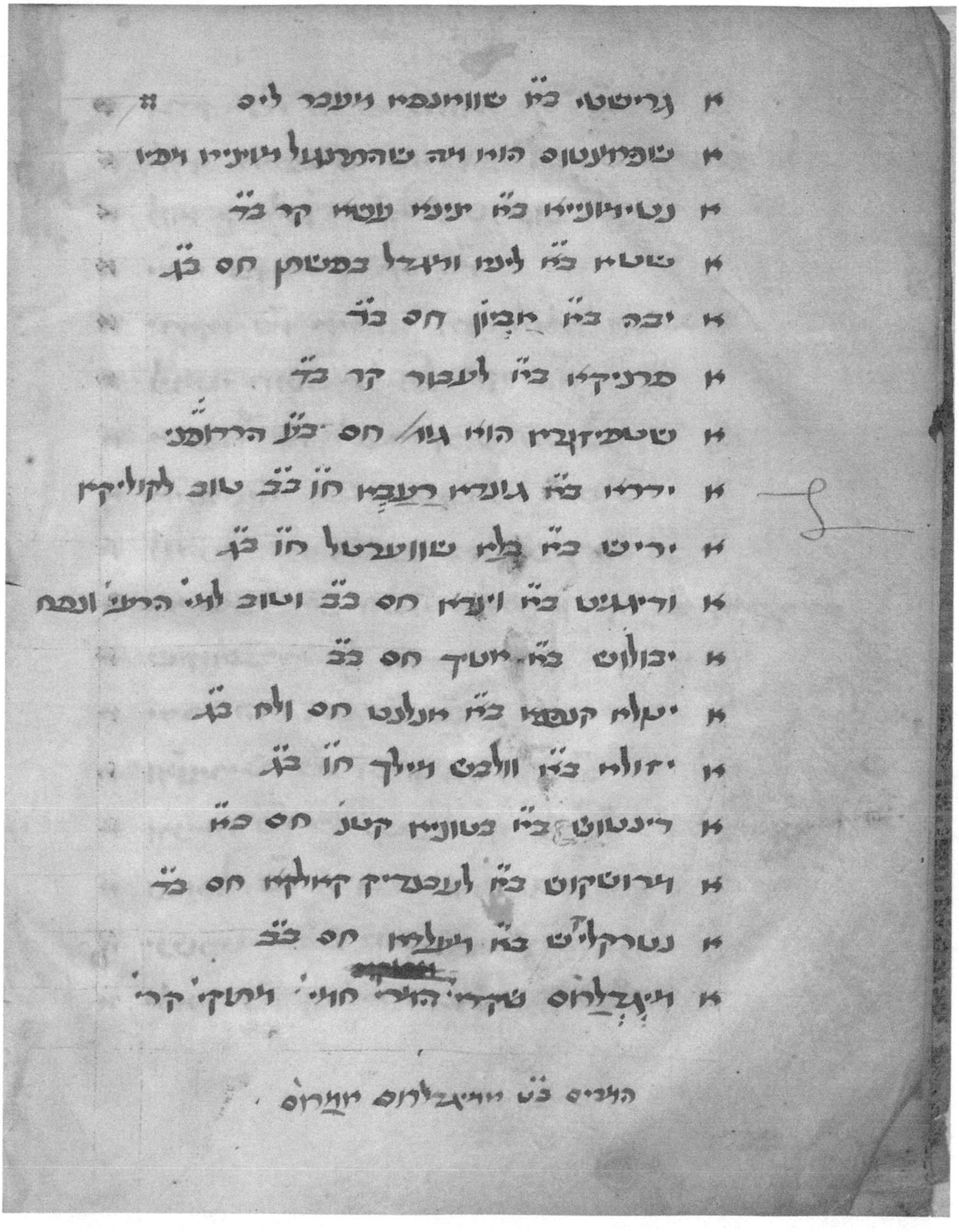
א גריסטו בה"ו שוומנפיו מעמר ליפ
א שפרועטופ הוא מה שהתרגל מעיירו ומפו
א נטימוניירו בה"ו יוינוו עטוו קר בד"ר
א שטיו בה"ו לינו ורגל במשתן חם בג"
א יבה בה"ו חבון חם בד"ר
א פרניקיו בה"ו לעבור קר בד"ר
א שטמידקין הוא גיר חם בע' הרדופני
א ירדיו בה"ו גונדיו רעבו חו בב' טוב לקוליקו
א יריש בה"ו בלח שוועדטל חו בג"
א וריגניט בה"ו ויגדיו חם בב' וטוב לוי' הרע' ונפח
א יבוליש בה"ו מטך חם בב"
א יעולה קנבאו בה"ו מנלגט חם ולח בג"
א ידולה בה"ו וולבט מילך חו בג"
א ריגנוט בה"ו בטוניו קטן חם בה"ו
א מרושקוט בה"ו לעבדריך קאולקו חם בד"ר
א נטרקליש בה"ו מעלתו חם בב"
א מיגדלוס שקדי' הרי' חוי' מתוק' קר'

הנוים בט מיגדלוס מקרוס

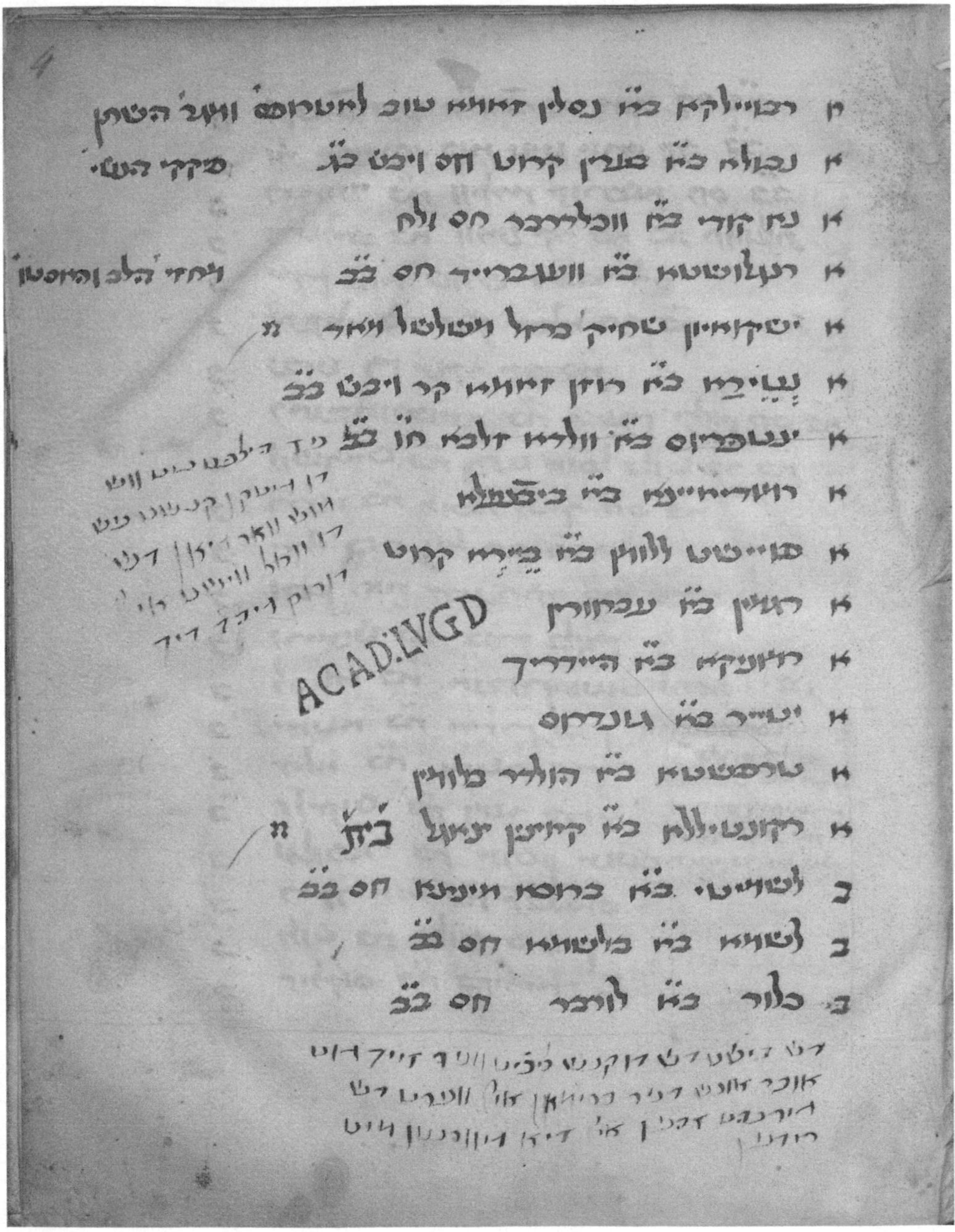
ACAD.LVGD

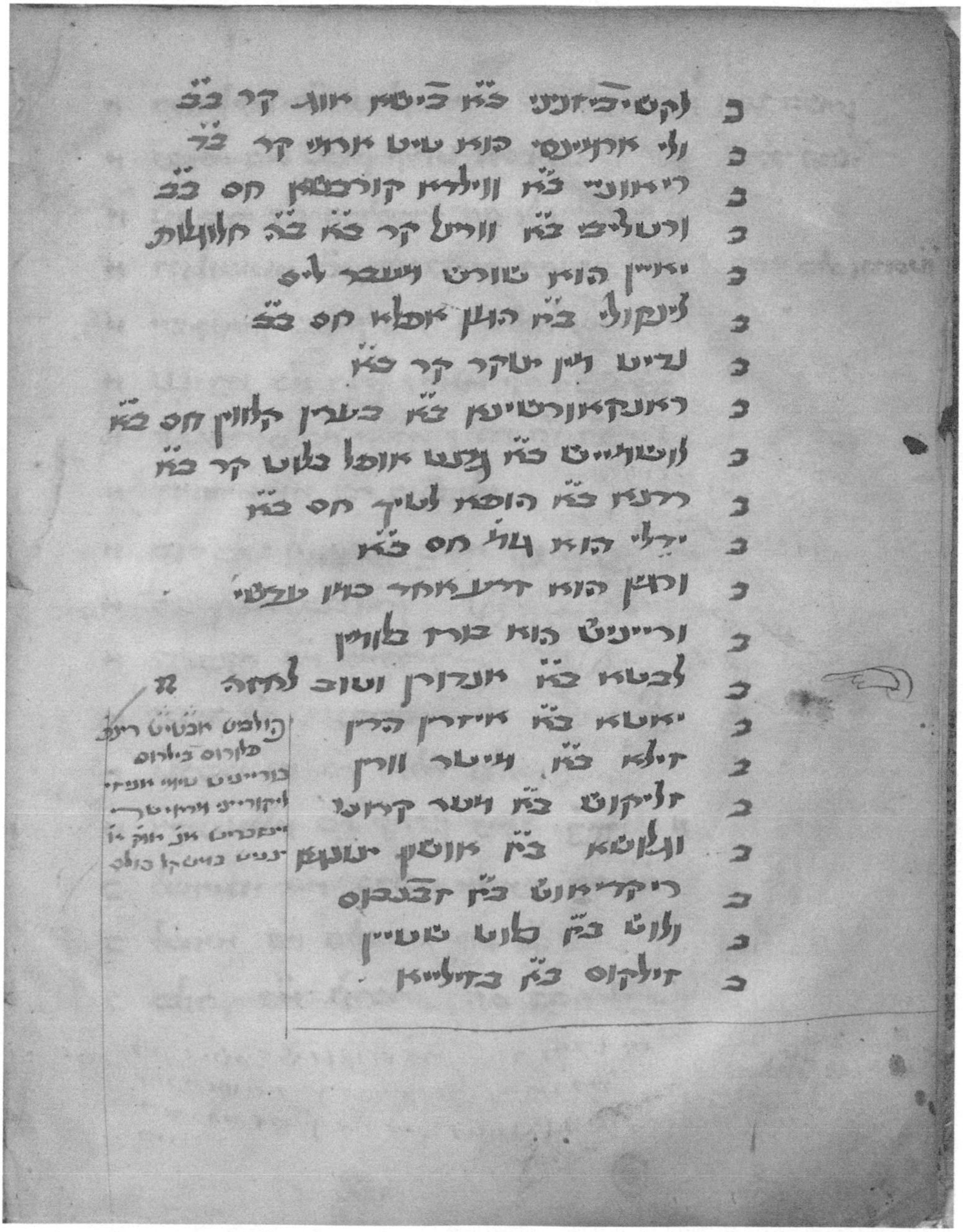

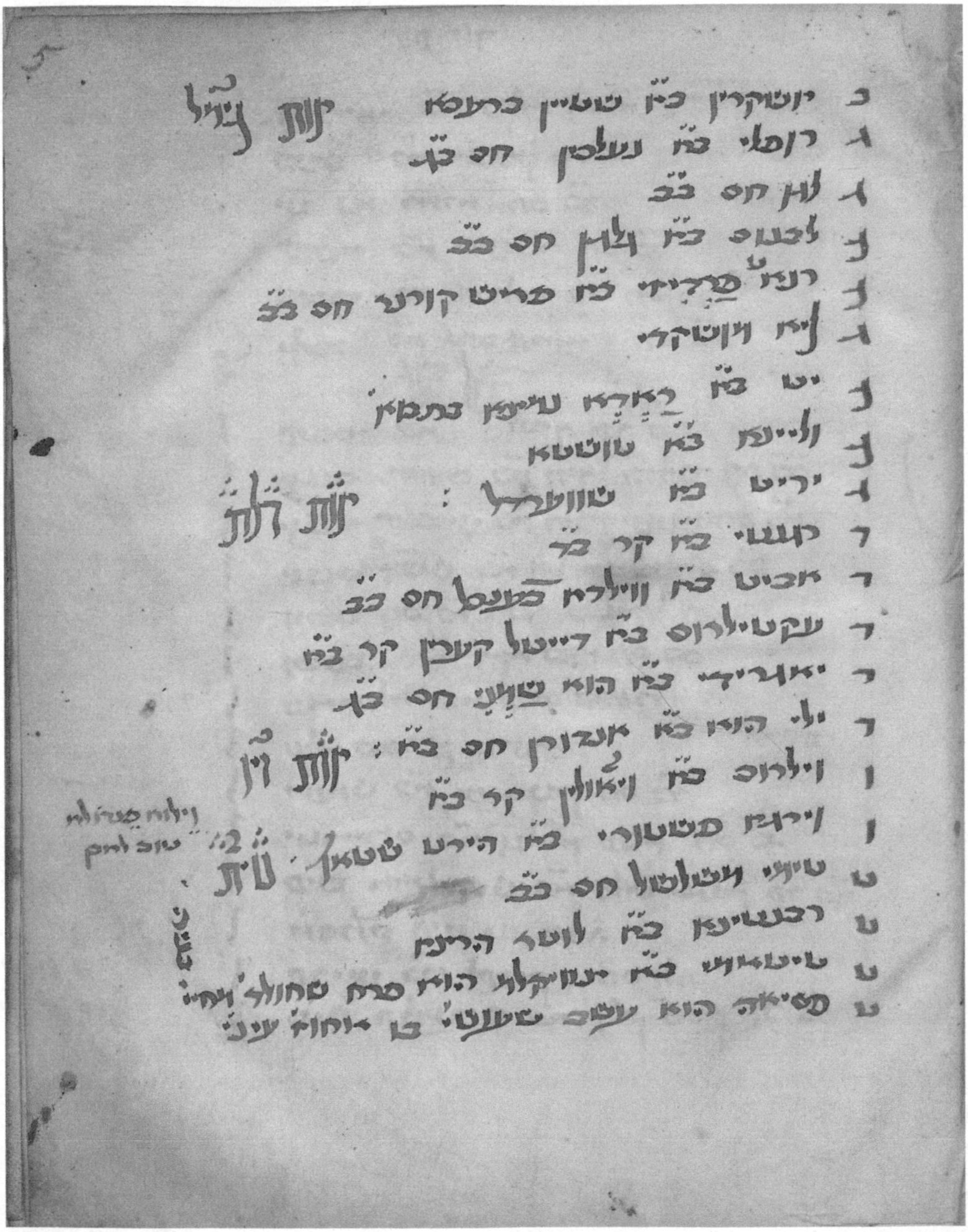

ב יושקרין בת״ שטיין ברעפא יזת נז״ל
ג רעפלי בת״ נעלכין חס בב״
ג לון חס בב״
ד לבונה בת״ בלין חס בב״
ד רנה פרידי בת״ פרנט קורנר חס בב״
ג ניה וושקרי
ד יטו בת״ ראורא עייפא בתמן
ד ולייגא בת״ טושטא
ג יריט בת״ שוועדרל : יזת דלת
ר מששי בת״ קר בת״
ר אביט בת״ ווילרא מענטל חס בב״
ר עקטילרוס בת״ דייטל קעבן קר בת״
ר יאוריזי בת״ הוא שמעי חס בג״
ר ילי הורו בת״ אנדורן חס בת״ :
ו וילרוב בת״ ניאולין קר בת״ יזת וין
ו וירבא פטטורי בת״ הירט שטאל
ט טיזי מטולטול חס בב״ עית
ט רבשייגא בת״ לוטר הריגא
ט טיטואיש בת״ יעזיקלא הוא פרח שחולי ומי׳
ט פסיאה הוא עשב שעניי בו אחוזי עני׳

וילוח מרולא
בג״ טוב וחם

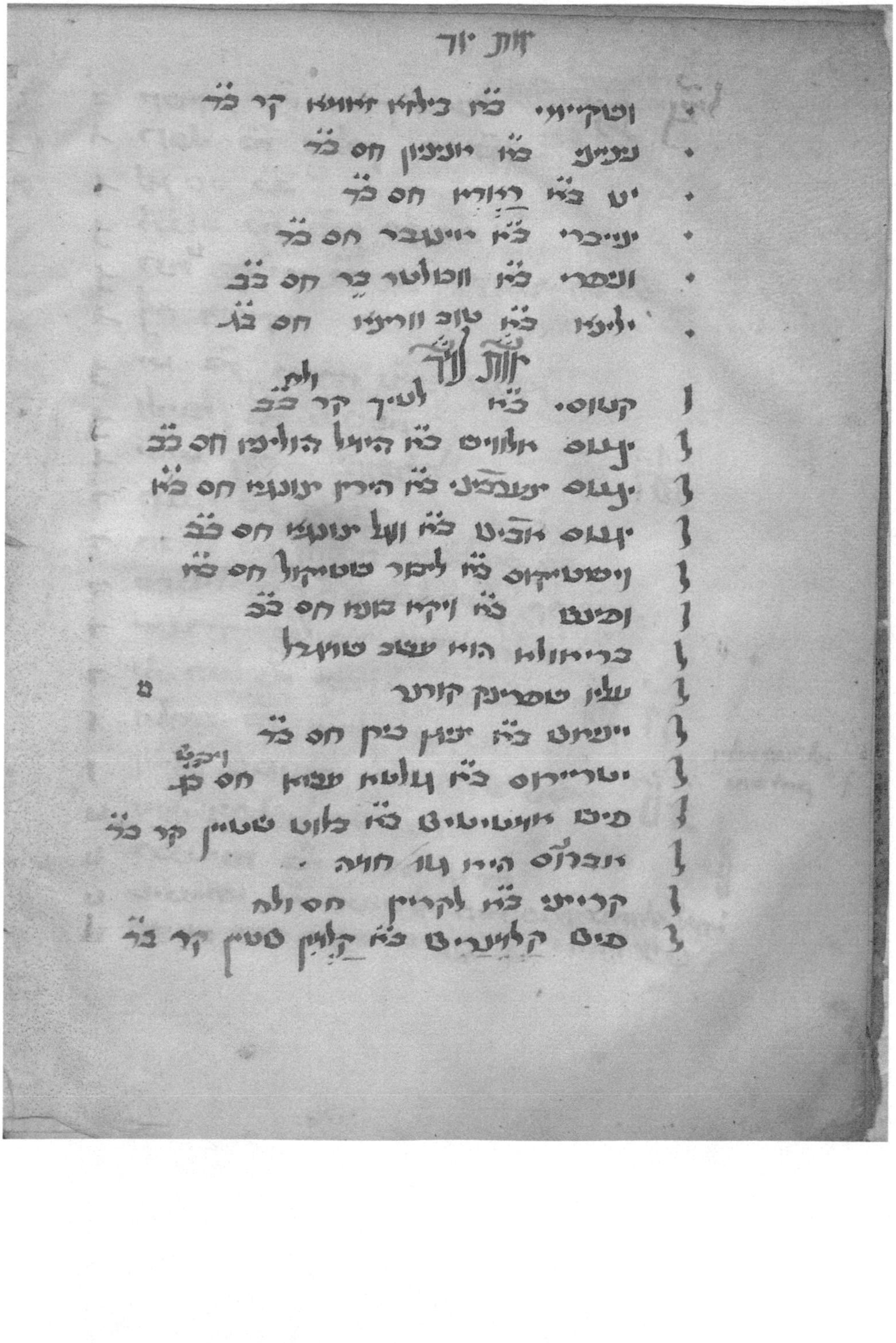

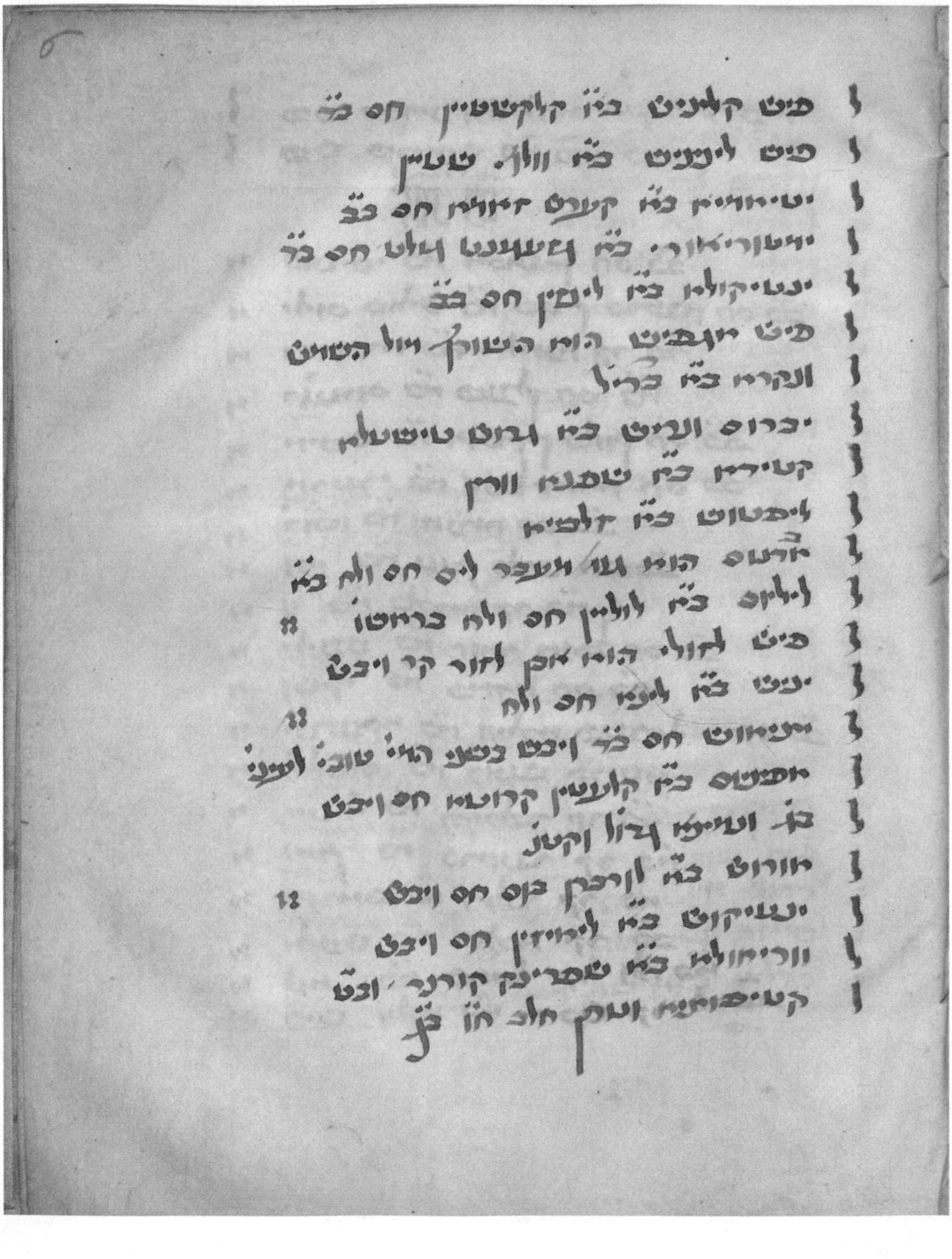
6
פיט קלאניט בלע״ קוקשטיין חם כ״ר
פיט לאנגניט בלע״ וואל. שטיין
יטיאודיין בלע״ קערס יאודין חם כ״ב
יאשטוריאורי בלע״ גשענגט אלט חם כ״ד
ינטיקולא בלע״ לימין חם כ״ב
פיט אנגביט הוא השוהם ואל השוהם
ונקרא בלע״ ברי״ל
יברוס ובריט בלע״ גרוט טישטלא
קטירין בלע״ שפנא וורן
לימטוט בלע״ קלמינ
אורטוס הוא גזו מעבר לים חם ולח בלע״
לאליא בלע״ לולין חם ולח ברמשו׳
11 פיט לאולי הוא אבן לדור קר ויבש
ינגיט בלע״ לאגני חם ולח
22 אנגיאוט חם כ״ר ויבש במעי האי׳ טוב׳ למעי׳
אמפטוס בלע״ קוענין קרוטא חם ויבש
בג׳ ושיאג גדול וקטן
אורוט בלע״ ורפק בוס חם ויבש
12 ינשיקוט בלע״ לימוזין חם ויבש
ווריאולא בלע״ שפריגן קורנר ויב״ש
קטיפואשה ושק חלב חו״ בג׳

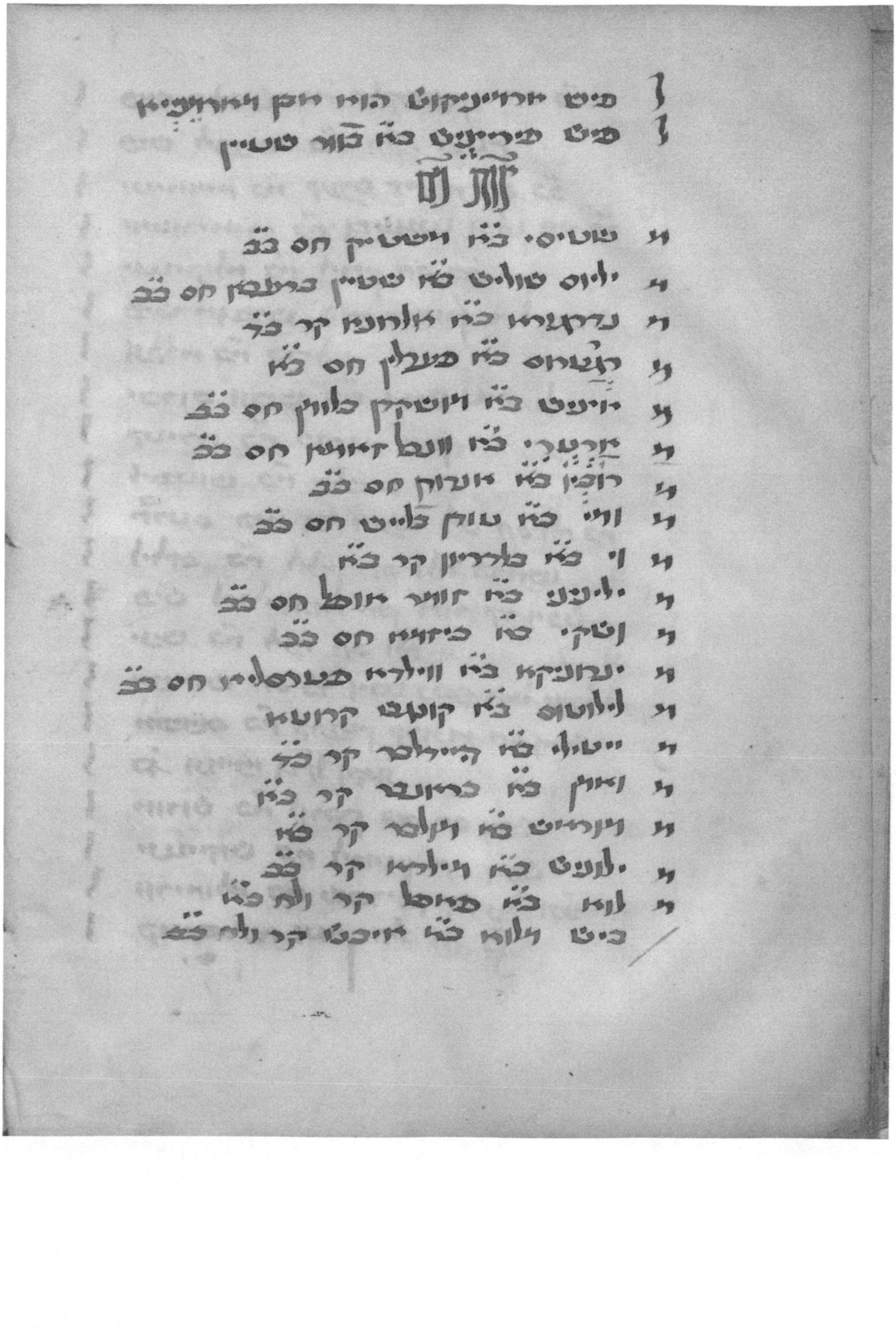

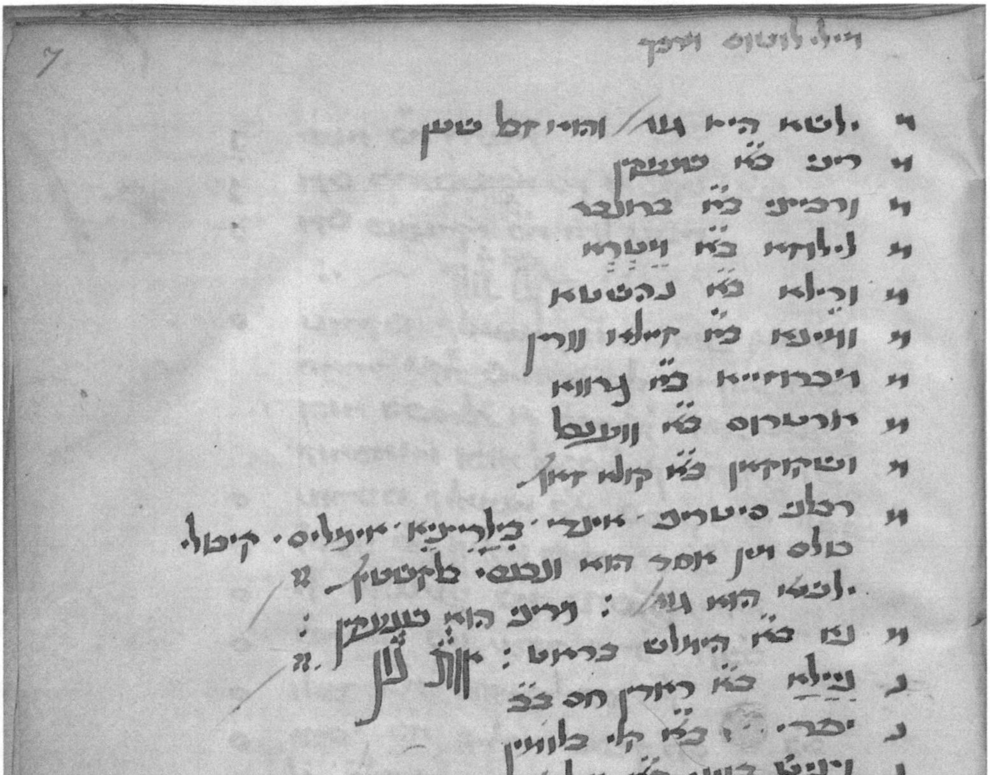

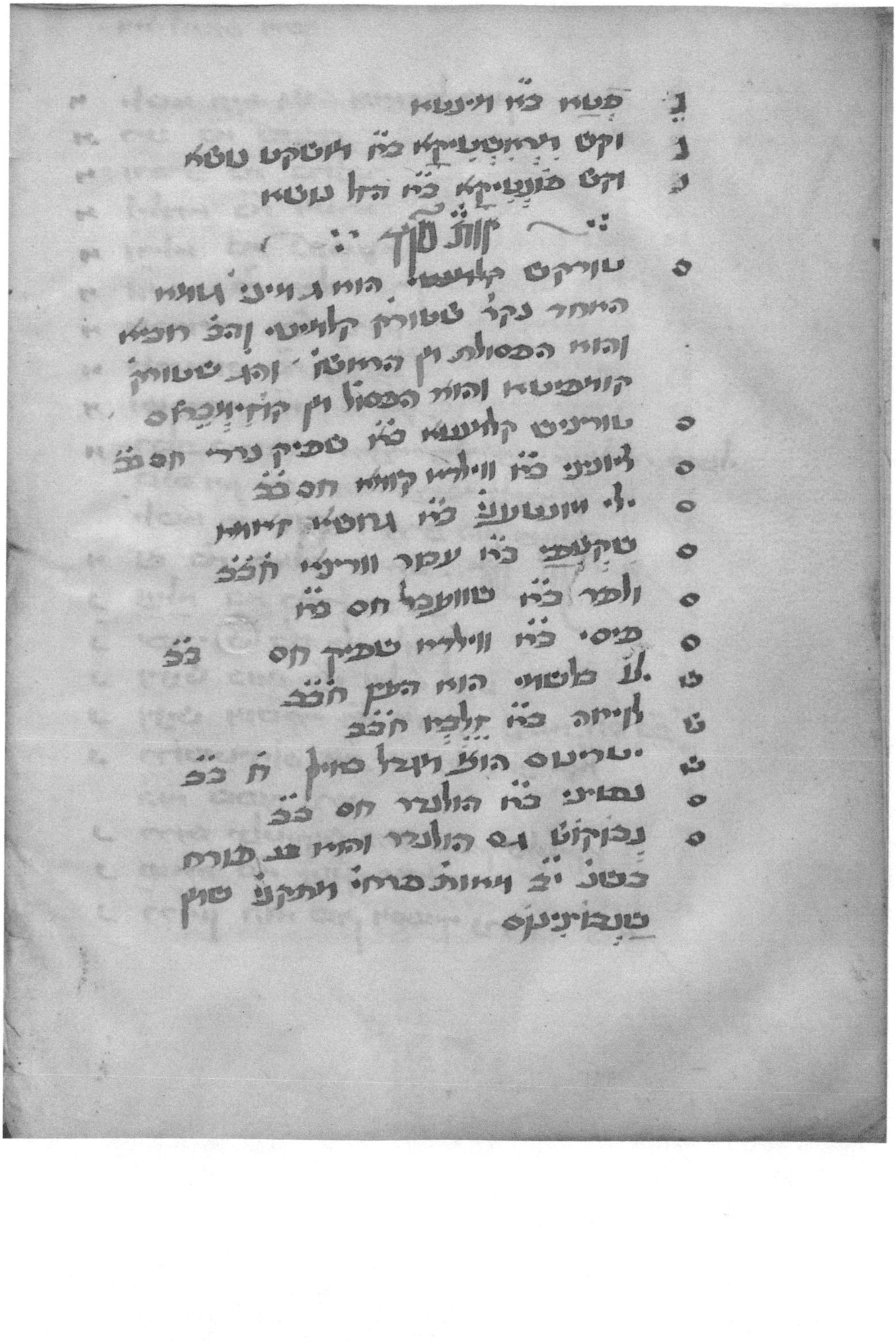

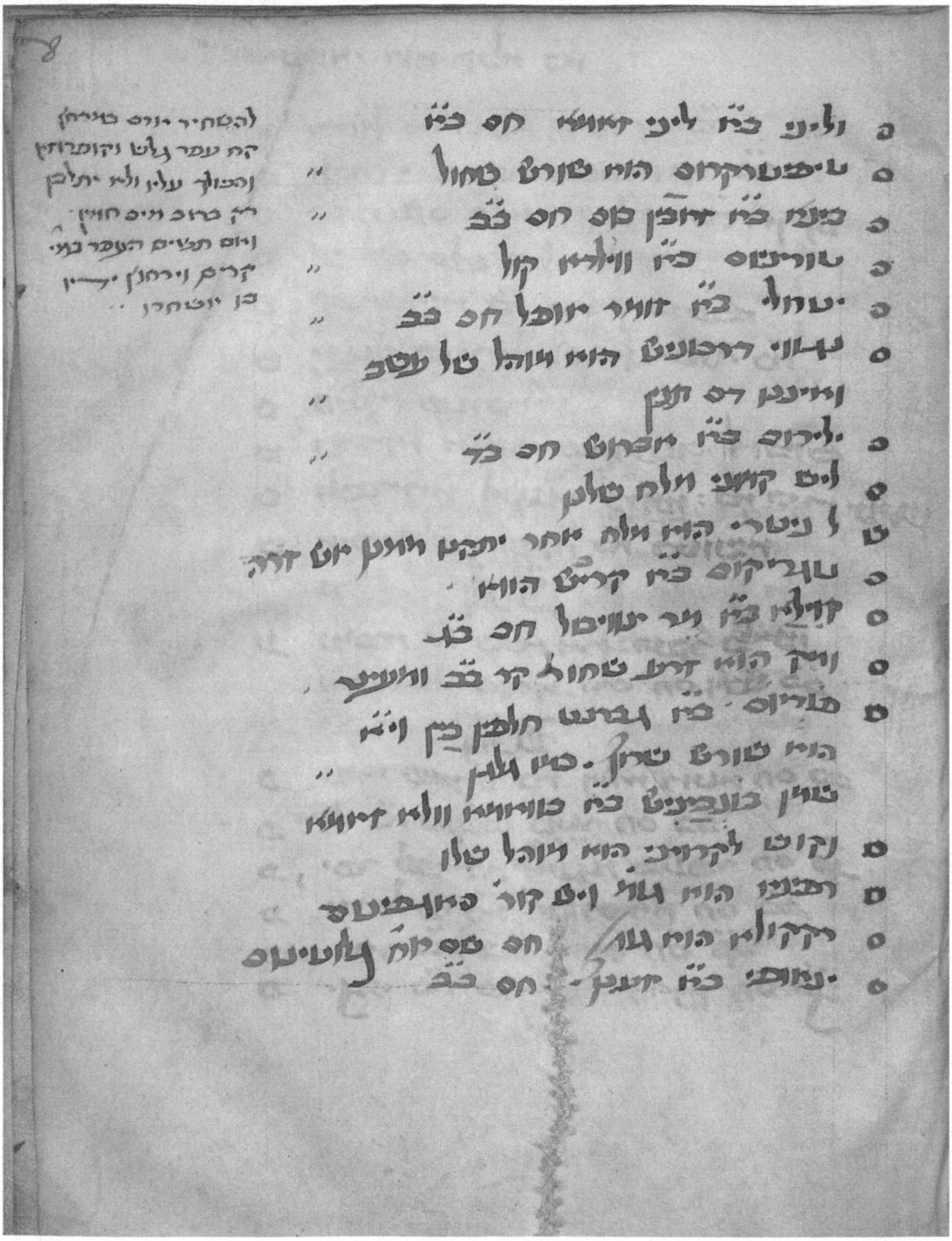

סיטוני הום קנלא כֹּ

ש מרוון כֹּ הוטיו וורמו קד כֹּ
ט ולטח כֹּ נהטא טאחו קד כֹּ
ט קוינטוס פליחה קולרוס כח וין קֹ
ט הם עלם טול חיק
ט קטימריין כֹּ טטיין כרטבא
ט יעקף פעורסליוס אנרסטי כֹּ
ט ווילחא מטוס לאן
ט נרקו אמורי פיקריעטוס רומק
ט ולטבריריו לטטוס יצרופו כֹּ היין יעמן
ט מידרוס ביטוונקד כֹּ בטוטקל

אוה לן

על עוטחו יה טוטו ורב הטקד כליטו
ויֹ טטולי טקרקנ הים חם ויטל כֹּ

אוה חה

מ נטעי פאנים כֹּ וילוי דוטח חם כֹּ
מ ול כֹּ נטלקן כלטיר חם כֹּ
מ יטר לטי כֹּ אישט בטבר חם קֹ
מ טורטלטו כֹּ טטרטילוא חם כֹּ
מ יטיר כֹּ כתט רוף חם קֹ
מ יעטי כֹּ טטח כא וורנן חם קֹ

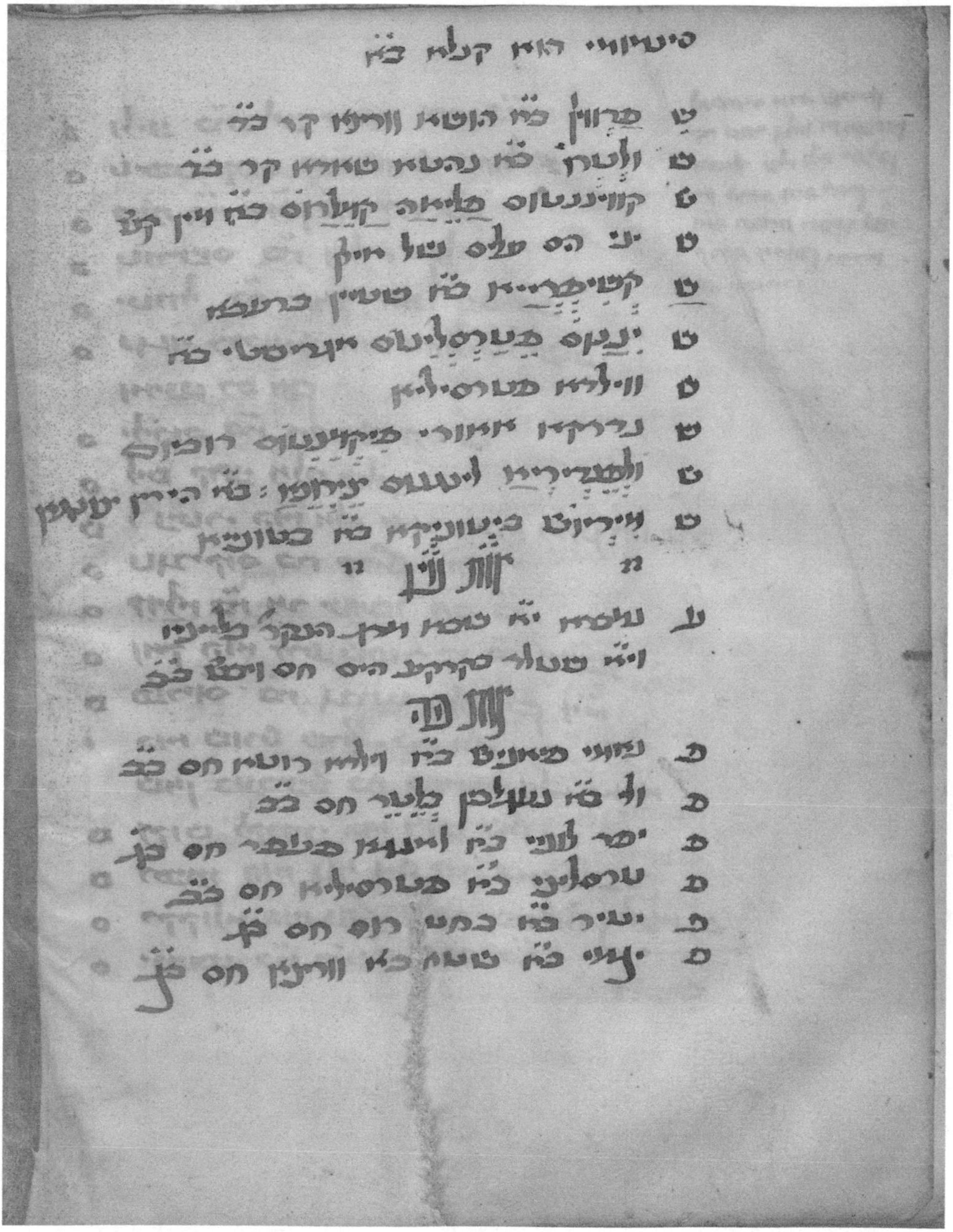

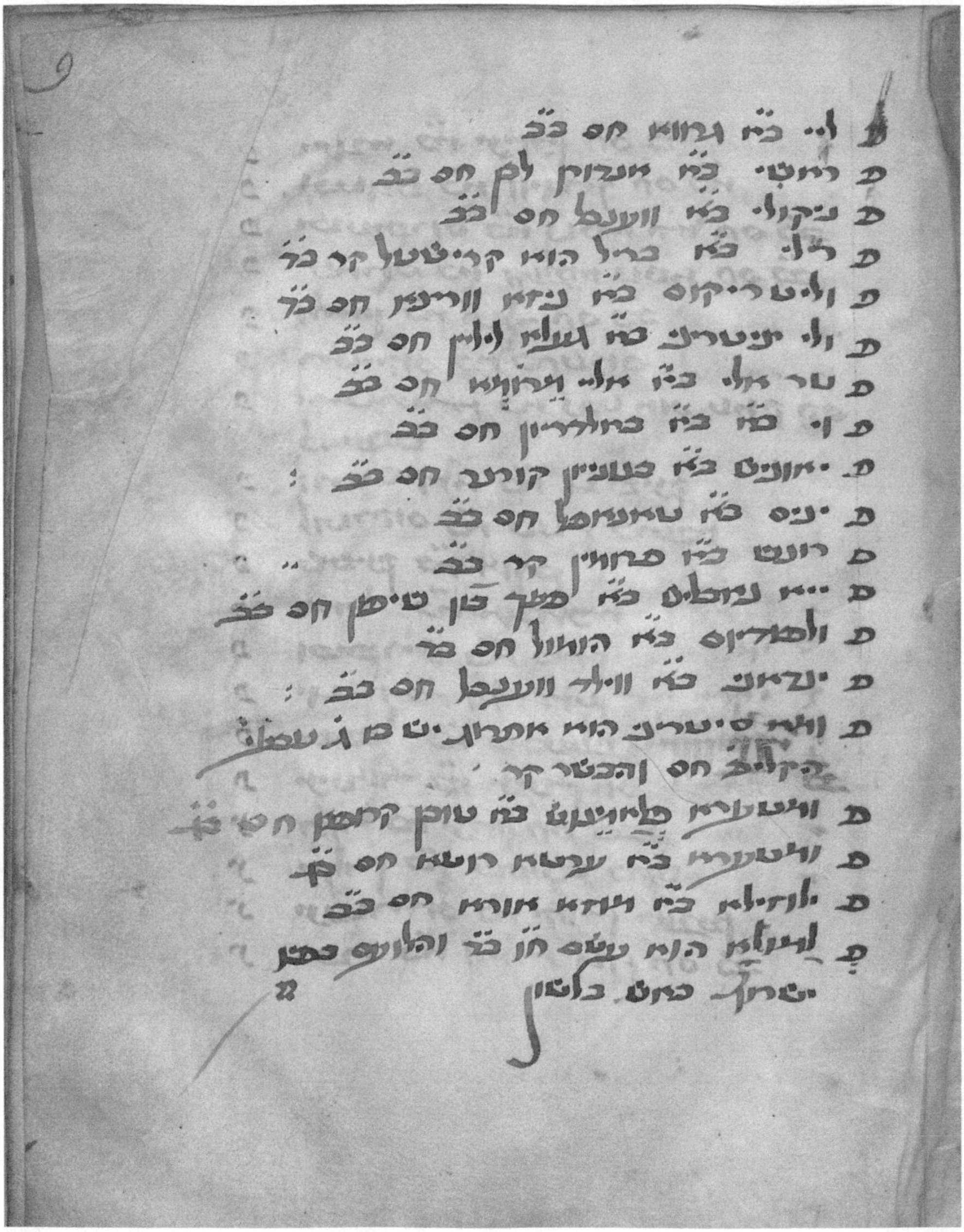

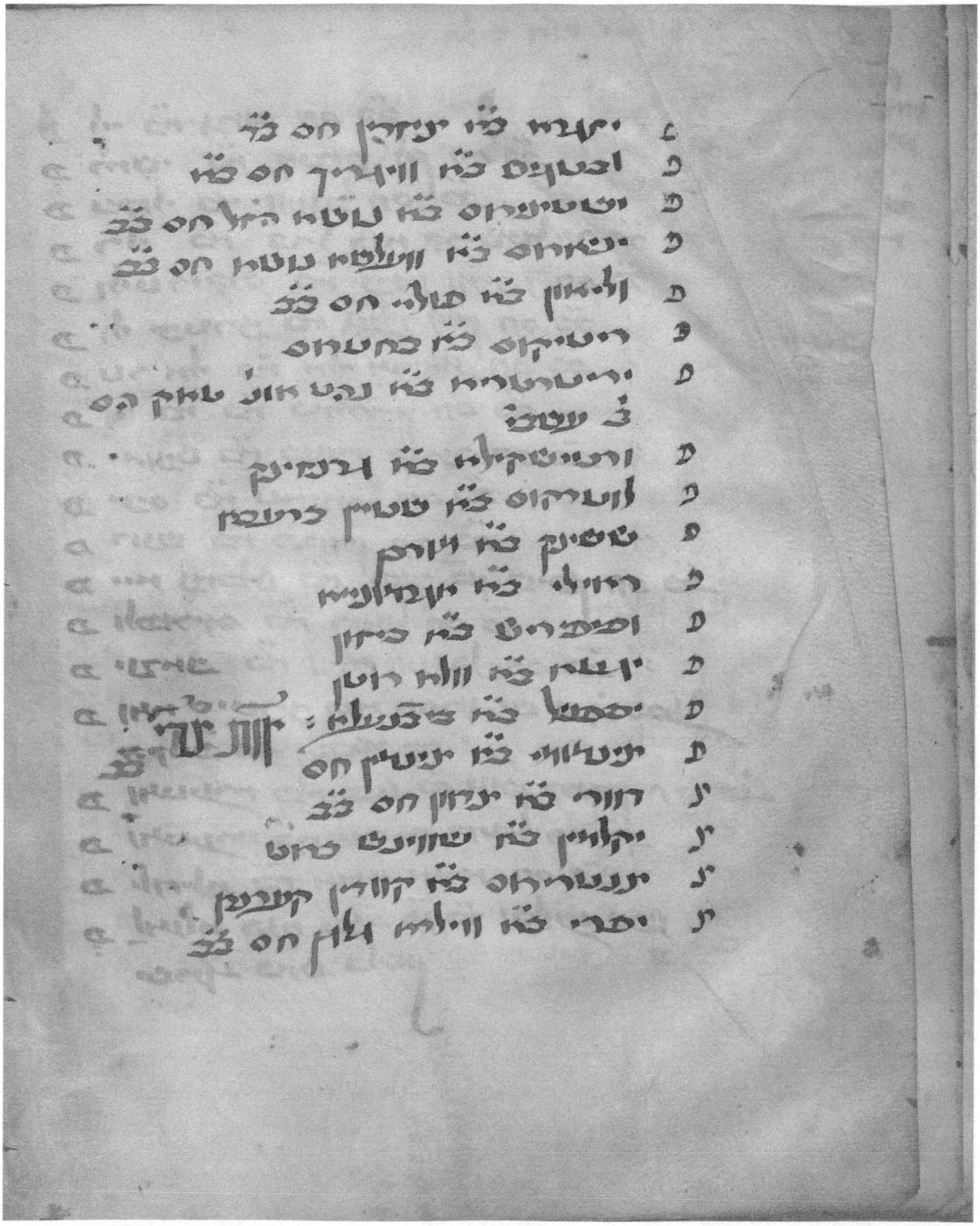

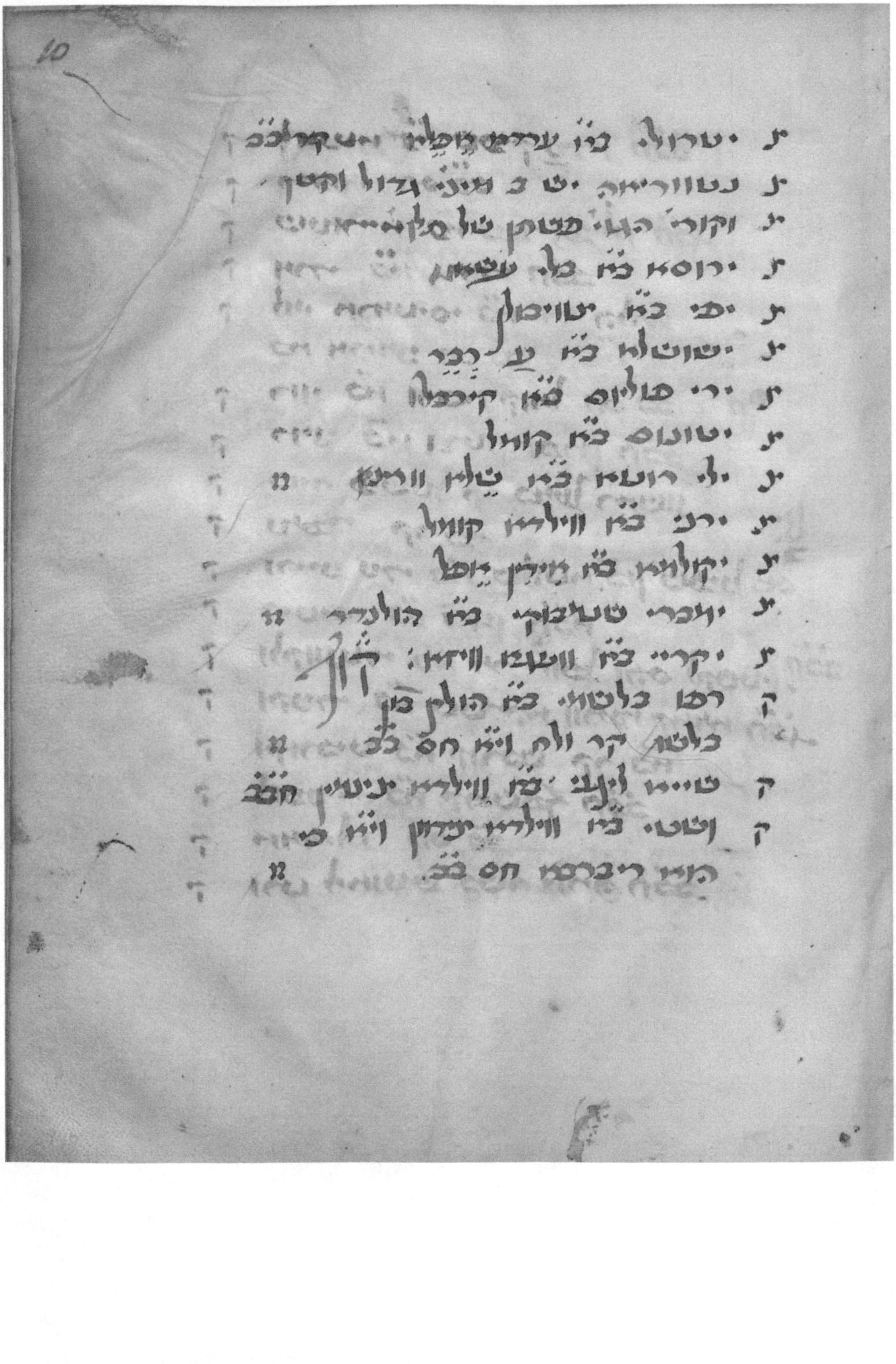

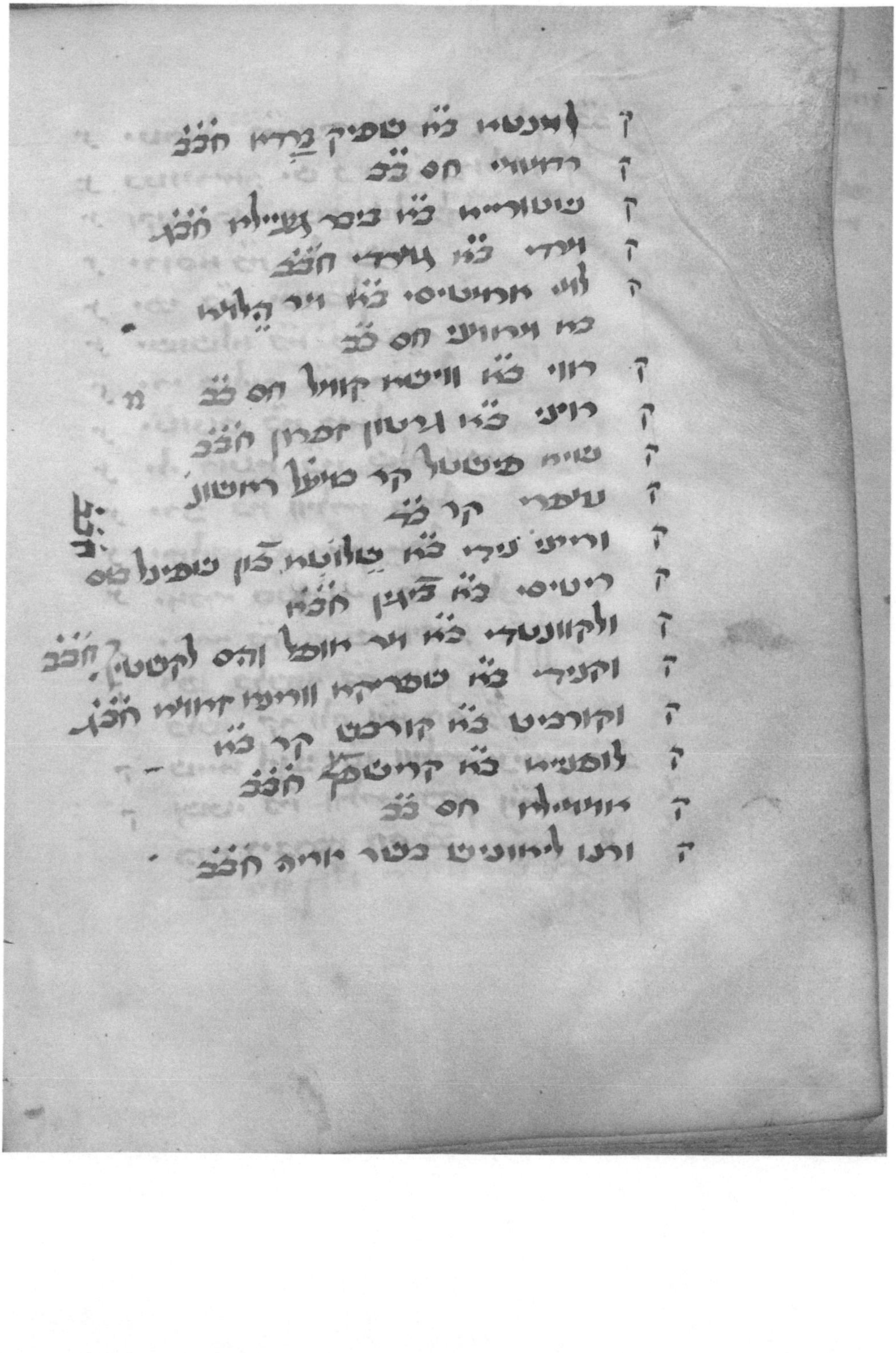

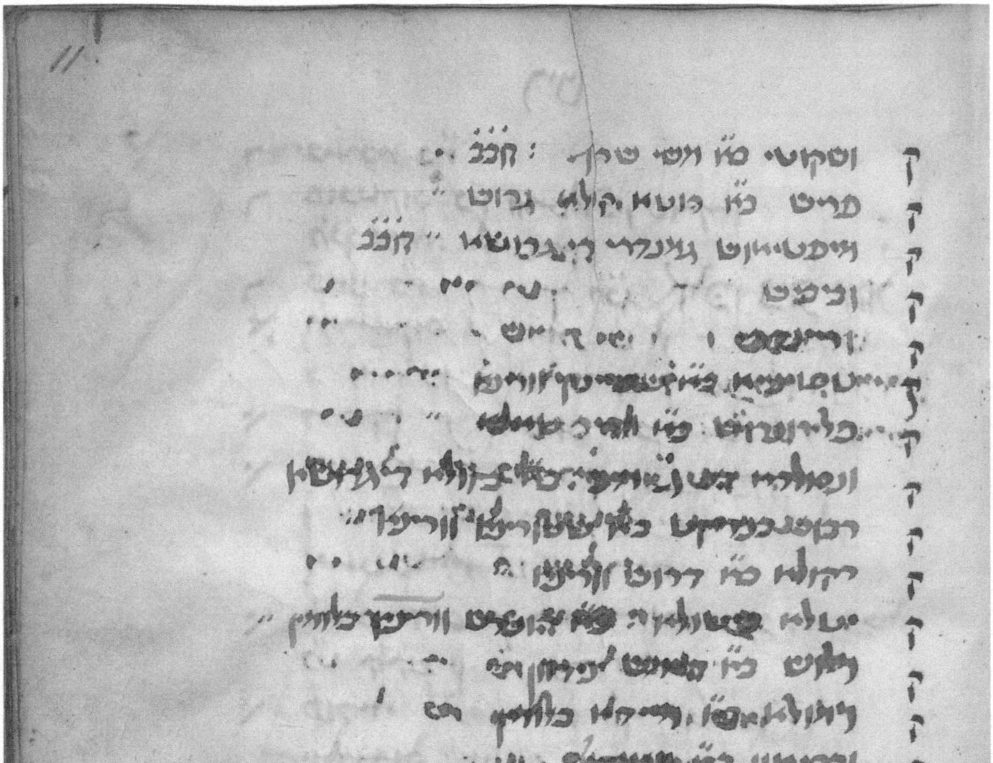

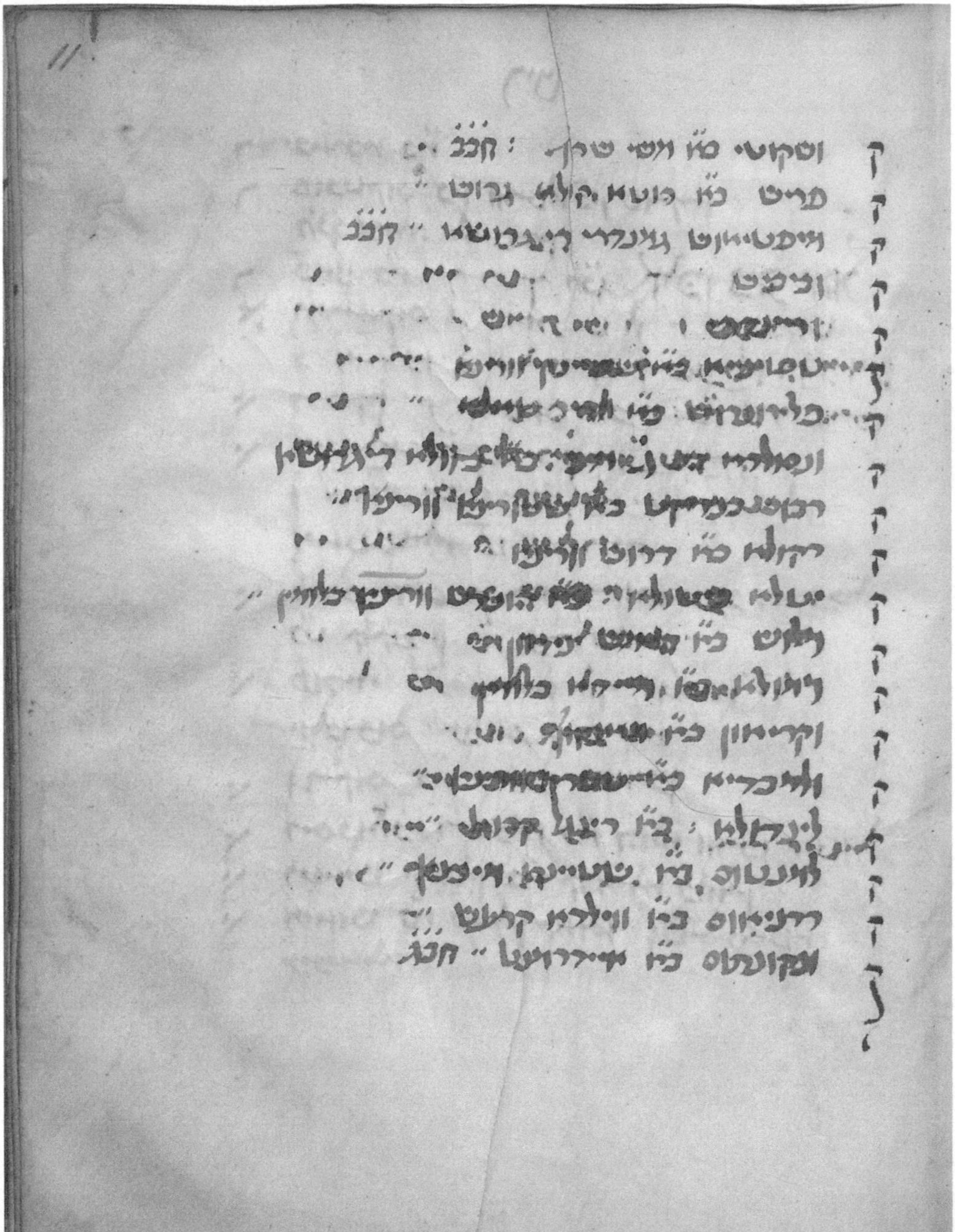

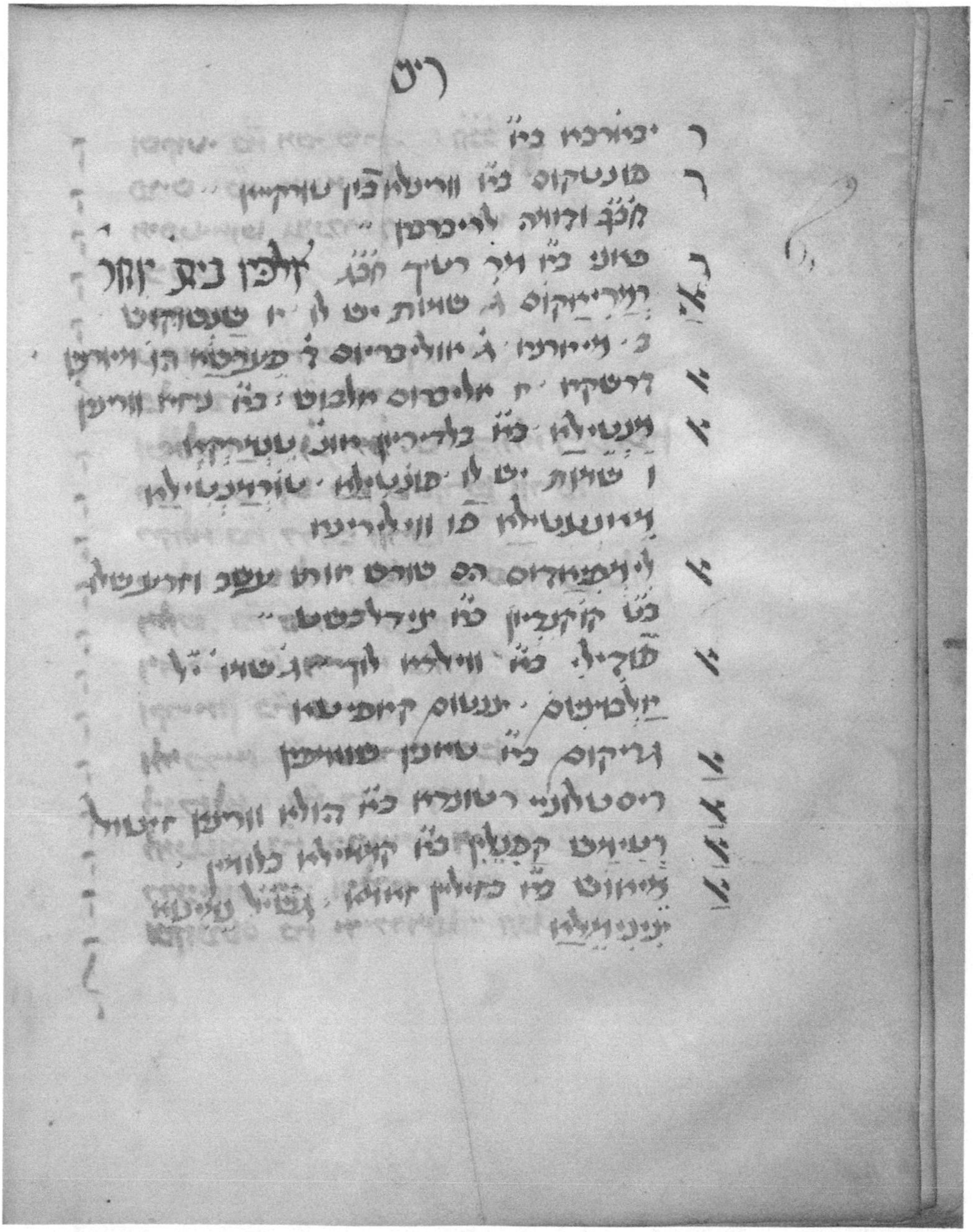

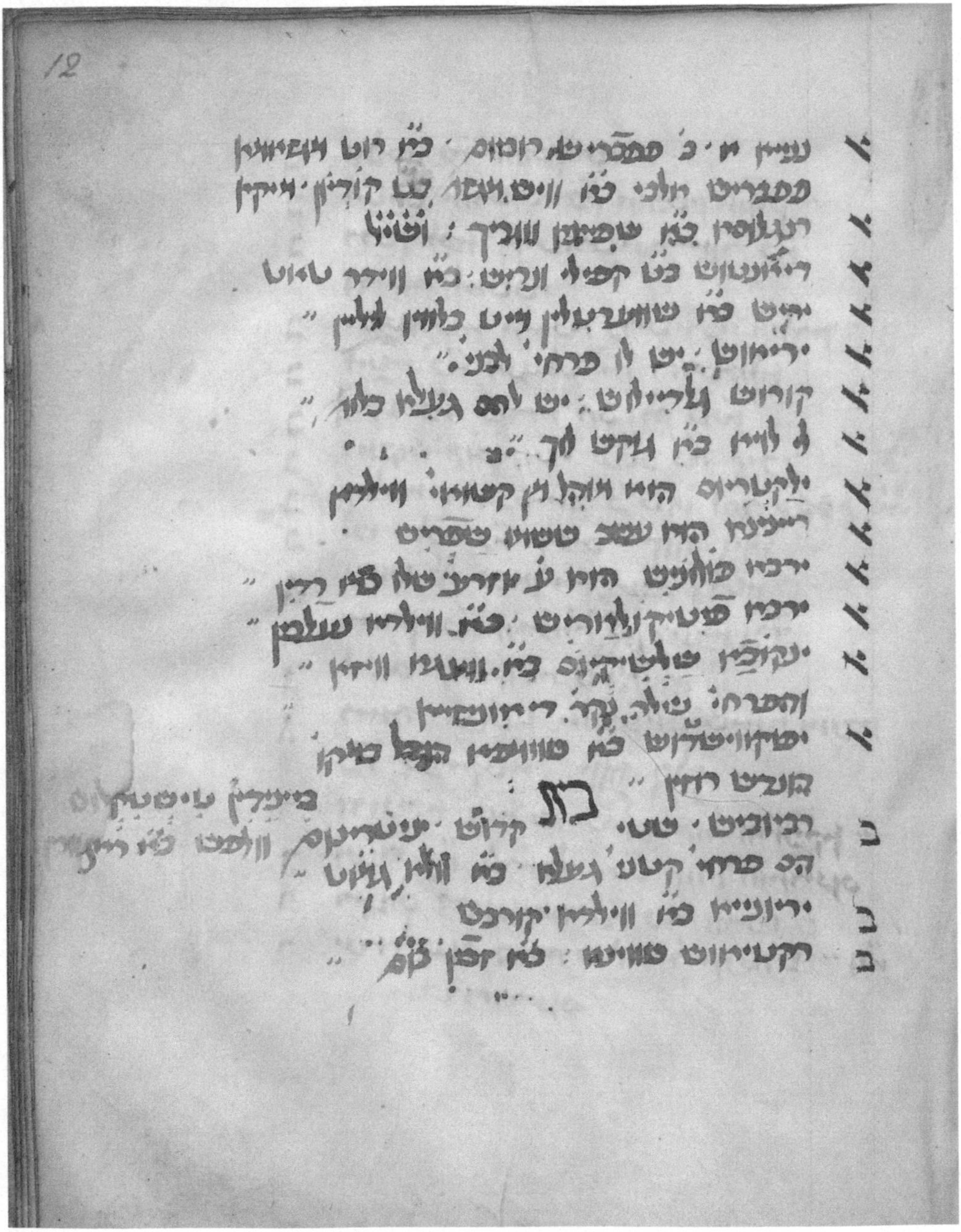

וקלשא מ יוהטין יעטט ב

לטיט יורטוט כ יוהטין מווטן כ

רעו לפו יעורטי מיוור כ ב
גרוטא לוטטי

יטטורטא יורפ כליטא כ מולדן ב
ליטא כ מעעוט יו רוטטקולא

ורגו מ כורחו חס ולח טי ב
חנקוט קושקוטי עטוב כ חידי

חילוקי רחעטיוה כ טחן וחר עסד ב
יט ולמו כ יעט – זות גימן

נקוט כ זטרן יין רעטן גרטין א

רמיין כ וורעולא טן רעטו נרחן ג
לוקוט קוטקוטי כ חירן

רייה יוטלטו מוועיוה טיעו ונטן ג
כ טפיקטא – זות רלת

ורוניקא הוד טורט יטו קר וורוטקן ר
מעט כ לורטולי כ חוטי לוחחעם

רעולס רקנעטייה כ נטד וורטו ר
יערו ליעעם הפח טו עק יעטוט ר
רוזרעם

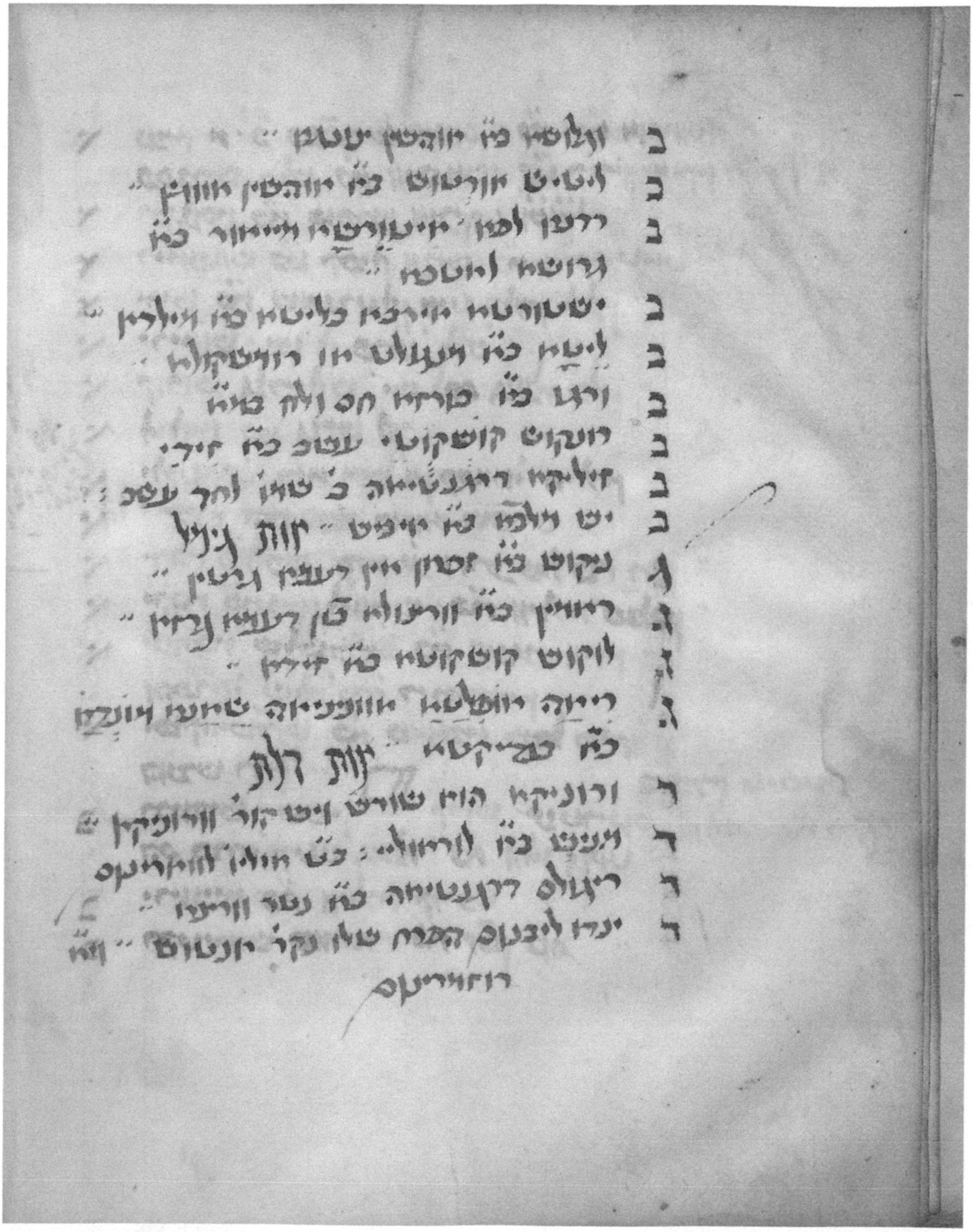

יפרין מוליפרין כׄו טטין וור ''   ה

רדיעו כׄו רוט הופן   ה

יעט זייקונט טולפורטו מא עשב   ה

זות הין   קעול הם גרעבע זערי '' זותוז   הכרו כׄו הוגרש   ה

מט ''   וירקמ פטטוריט כׄו וילאו קרטין ''   ו

ורוקרחא הויו עשב ''   ו

רמינו כׄו חיזר הרטיו '' זות דן   ו

יפיבריט כׄו דיינגבר ''   ז

יקעיא רוטא כׄו זוקי   ז

זות עזק   יטוורייא הויו טורט ''   ז

דרישקוט יׄע טהוו פרווין טוולמ ''   ט

יטחילטט יט כא וינו ה כׄו וולפמט וילך ''   ט

וערכיט הויו טארט ''   ט

פטיחא הויו טורט טיינגחיׄ כן כני יודא ''   ט

יחט המ נחט   ט

ורייענטילין הויו עשב ''   ט

זות זר   רטרוט כׄו וון טטין ''   ,

יעטתולי ייעטתי כׄו פרין   ל

זות לר   ,ל פיוווט כׄו וילדימ זלמו ''   ל

ליפיוט טפרוטיׄט כׄו טטין כרעמן זחוחו ''   ל

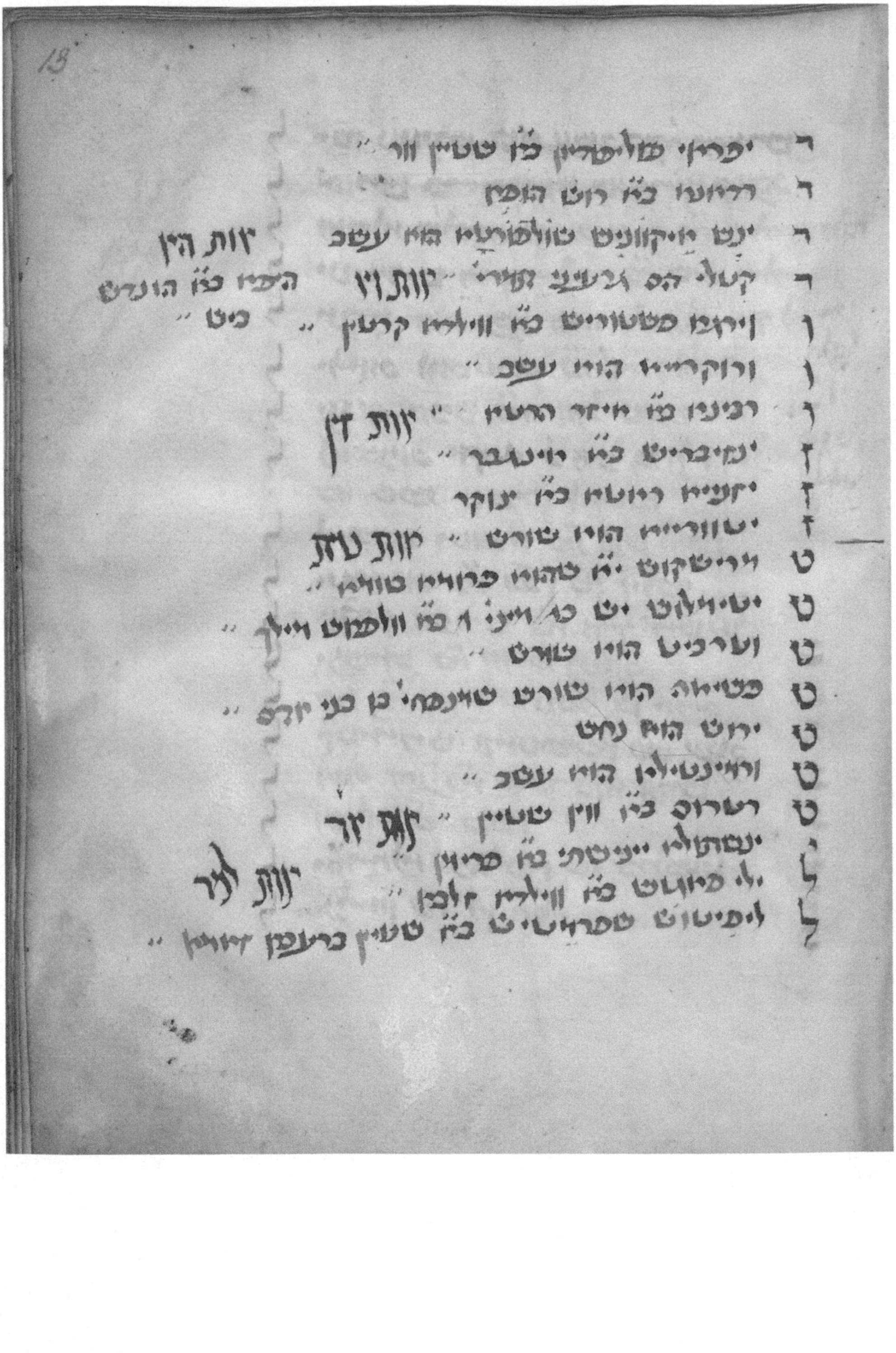

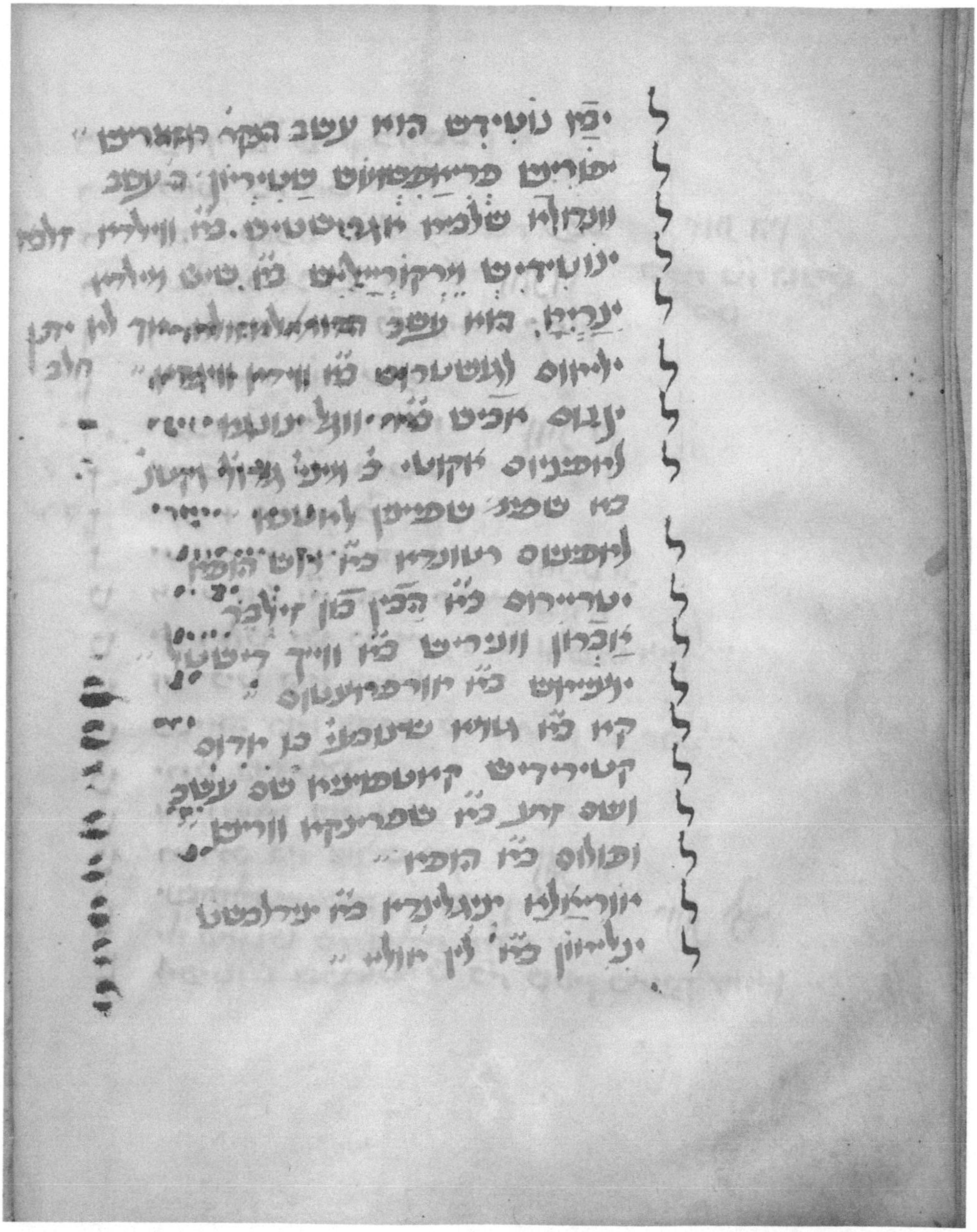

מ׳ ירטוש והחרע שׁל מרטליט והטין

נקר כּ׳ חולו מרטולי

מ׳ רוביוס פרעוס כּ׳ יונהין

מ׳ יעט כּ׳ וטטקרין בלוין

בּ׳ חבּחרטיקוס כּ׳ קול טהחתו לם

בּ׳ ולכולין ייוכרוחיין רימו כּ׳ גרוין

מ רטיויוס כווסו לוכיחו כ׳ נהט טרין

מ יקופוס יוק קוולין כּ׳ ווט מטירולי

מ נעטט כּ׳ יקן הוותך כרחל

מ יולו טילוויסטריין כּ׳ יופל יעלס יוט וולחין הקר הווערופו

מ ריקד יינטוטו כּ׳ חיילס יון פרעט

מ יוטיט הין עטר זר

מ יכטבילו כּ׳ מיטופט

מ וטקוט כּ׳ מירויין

מ וזי הורי פר חין הטייט מירוטו

מ יעיוס כּ׳ וטוטיס

מ וטיילייין הוי טוק עטוי לן כיחריין

מ ולטוריוס כּ׳ כו

מ רייוין וורקלי וונרט כּ׳ מיד יוורין

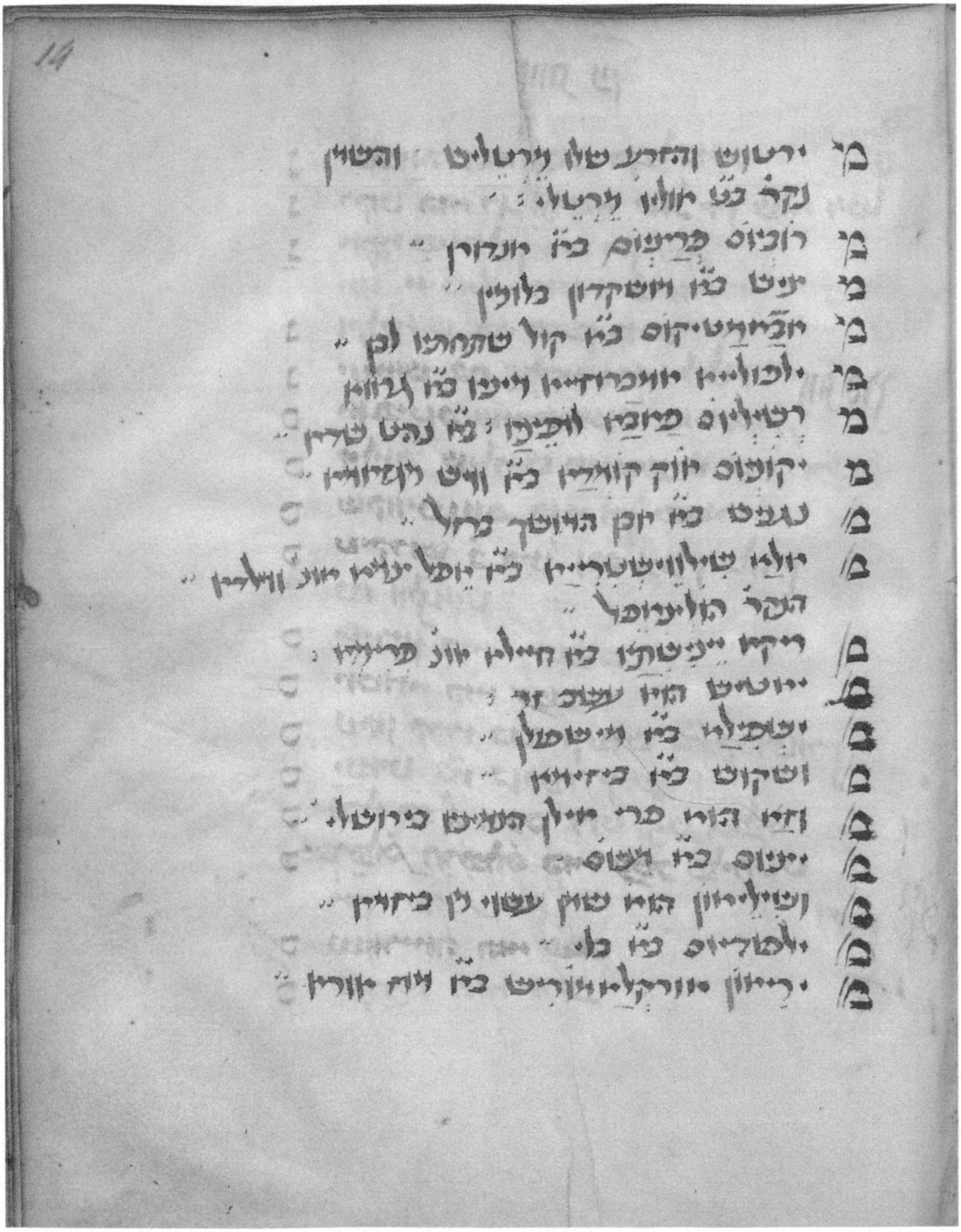

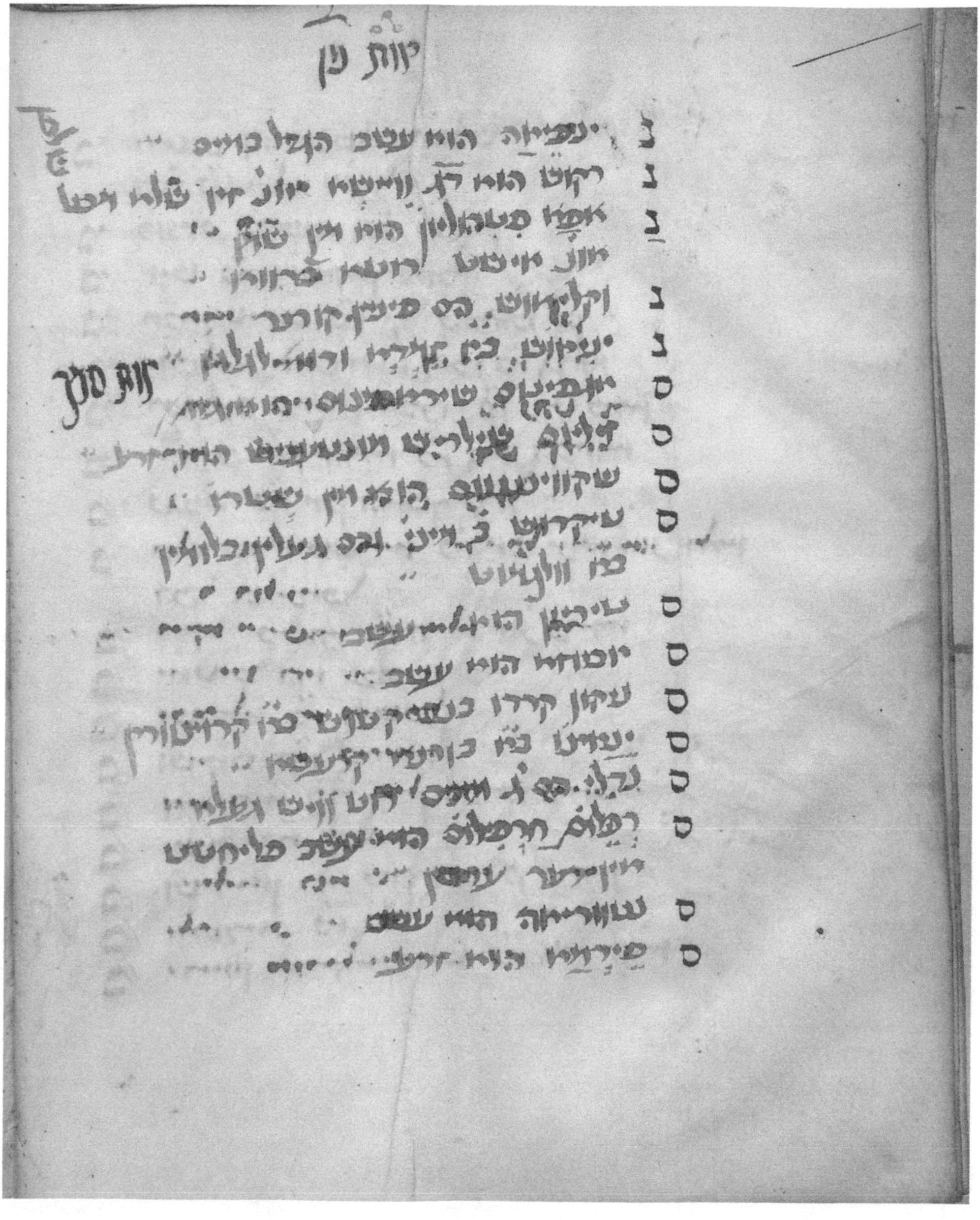

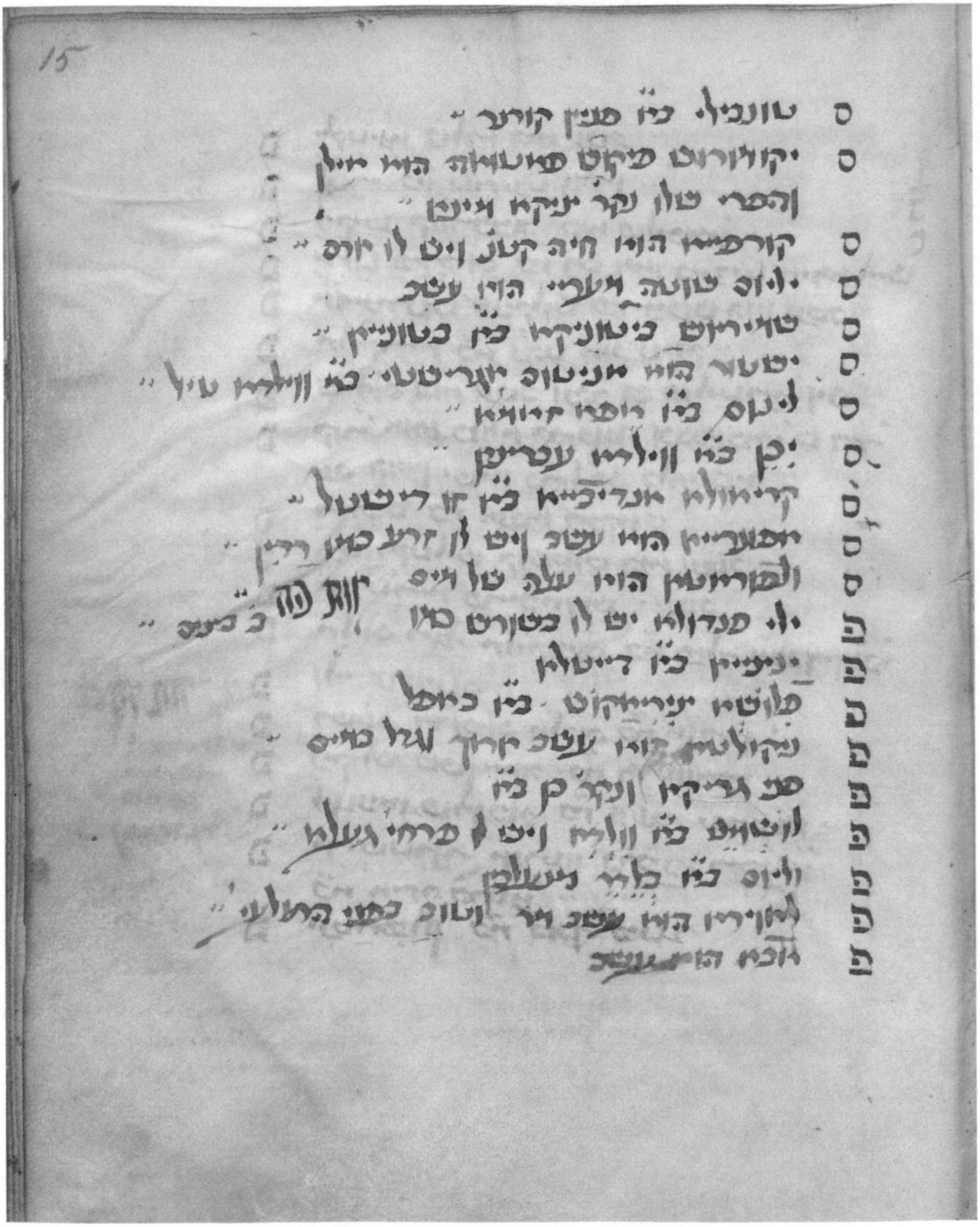

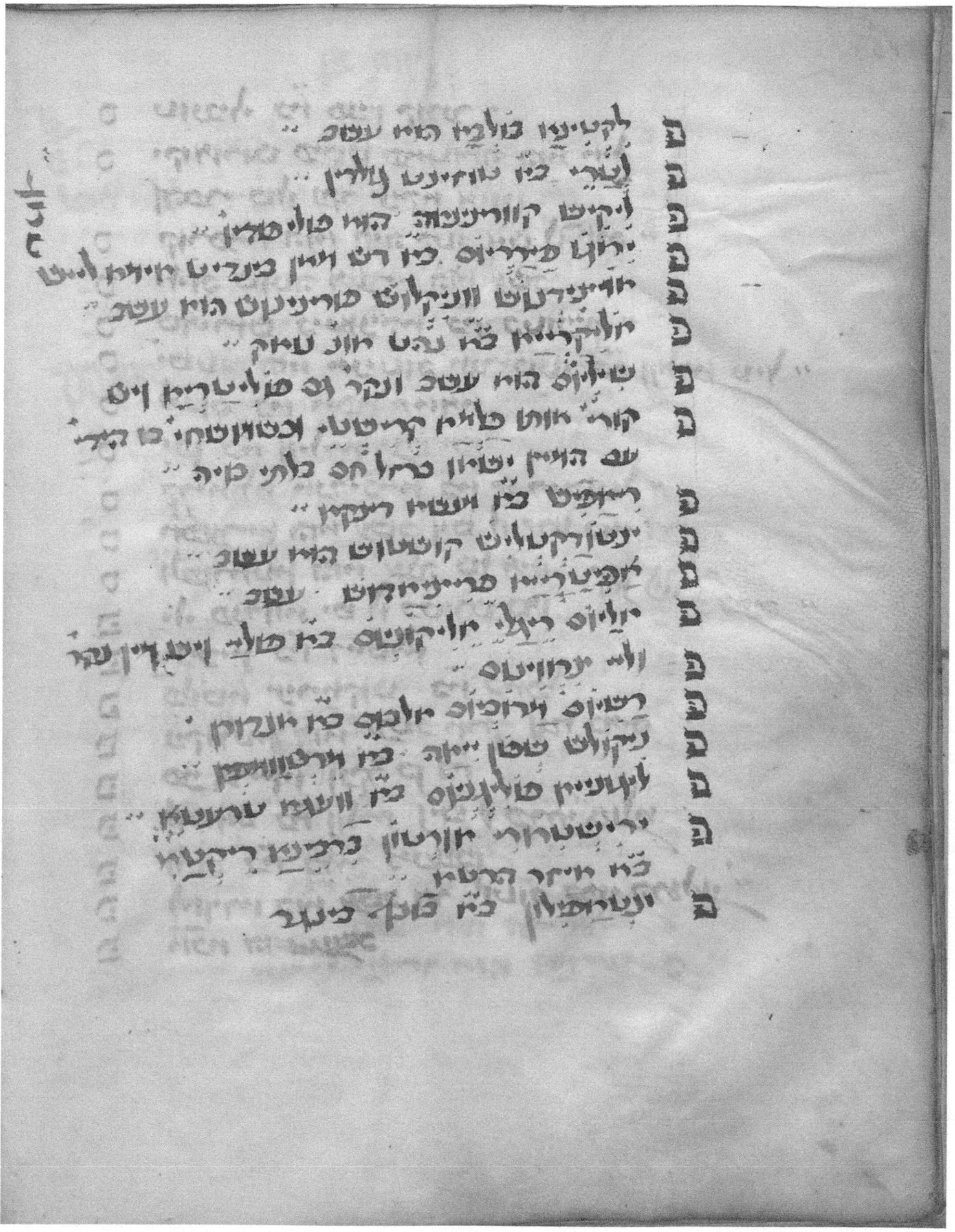

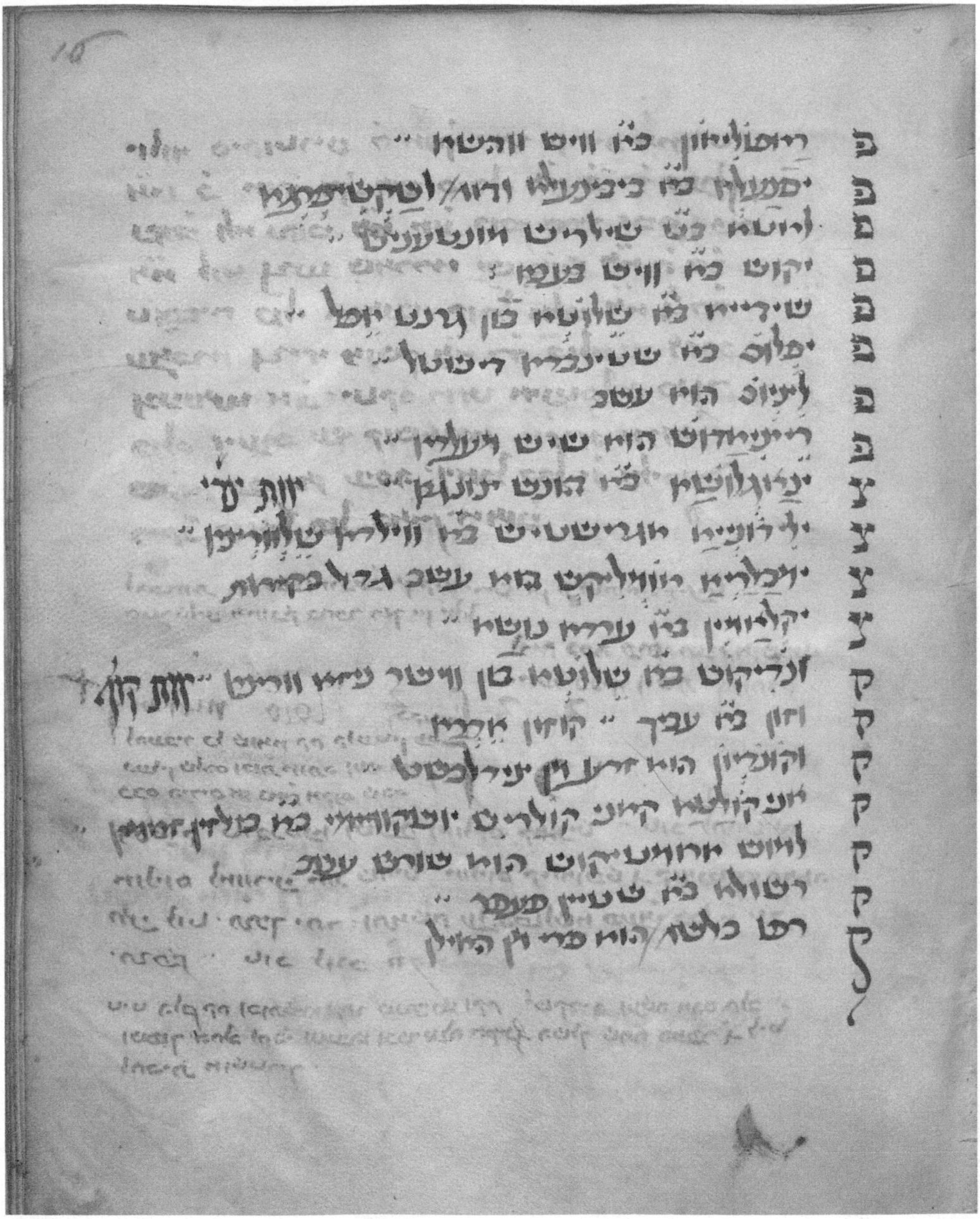

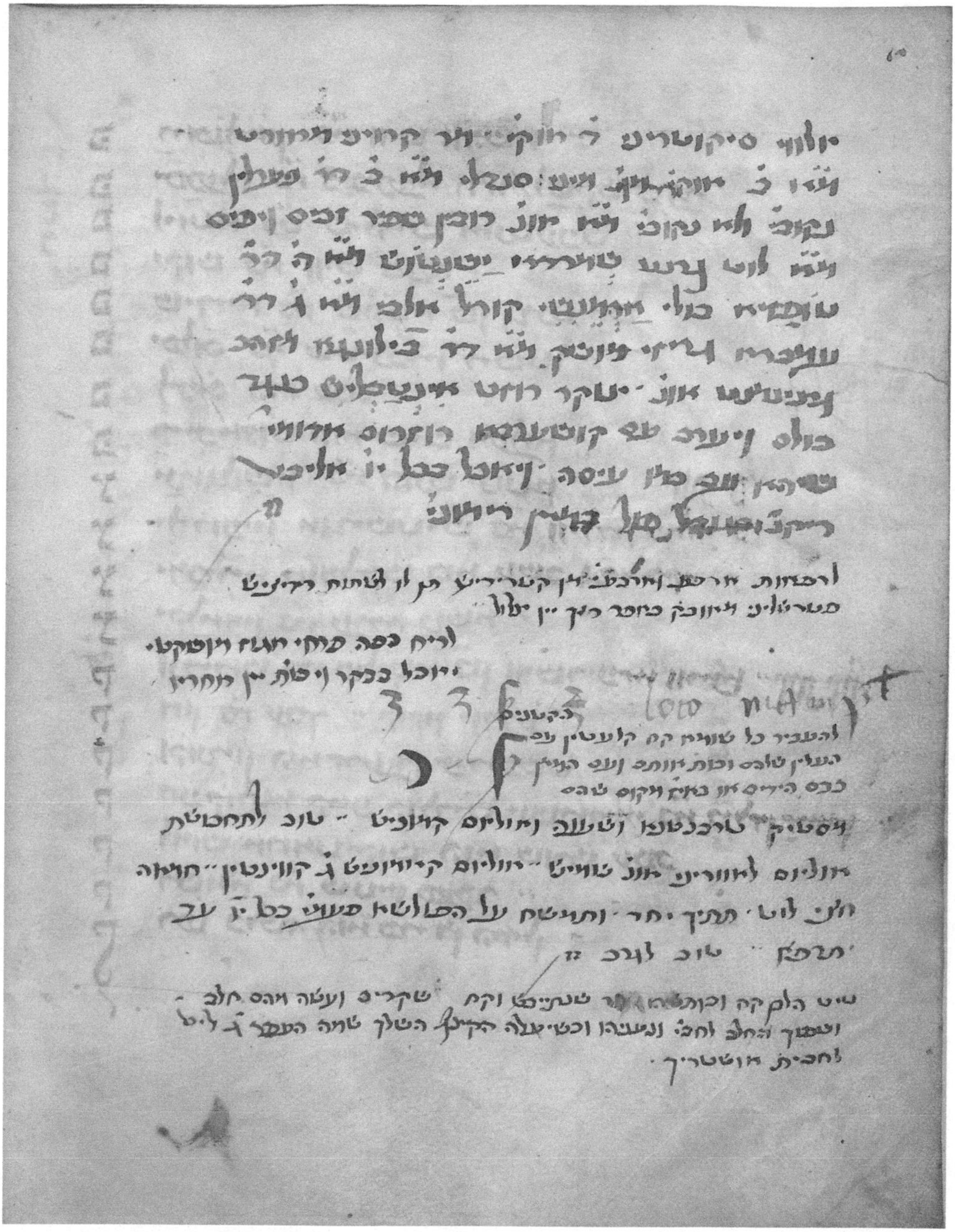

ק	קומע קרוו יוערישטי כו מע קומן
ק	רוטפורון פיט ירקמנס הוו עטכ כו היריט וט
ק	ריכולוגו בלוו פרובכמו וקרוע
ק	מיאקוו פשטיעקו כו וולוו וורהן
ק	רומיו כו יירהנעי ווט קול
ק	לועטו כו טוטין וינטו
ק	מיליוונעטו הוו עטכ טוערעיי כו חלכ
ק	רישטולו וו כ יעטוס גרעו כו הוערט קוע
ק	רוקוט וורעעולט כו זמן
ק	רוקוט וורטוענט כו וולוו זמן
ק	ועזוס ינקוטו כו עטכ טערומקו
ק	רפ מט פרוקטוט ידרי הם פר הגרו על עכך
ק	רווו וגרישטי כו וולוו וט קוו
ק	וטטוט יורטורוס כו גרטו וטכו
ק	וווקווועטר הו קוקורכטו וופמריו
ק	ורוס הוו כו טוריו ועוולי　　זות ריט
ר	ורן כו רוזו רוטוטטעו כו רחן וטר
ר	ווקטו רורן הוו טטיק יוע רוזן יוולו גריטטו
ר	וו הוו ריכרכו
ר	וט יעייקו כו כפלו לווין
ר	יטטו בוכט

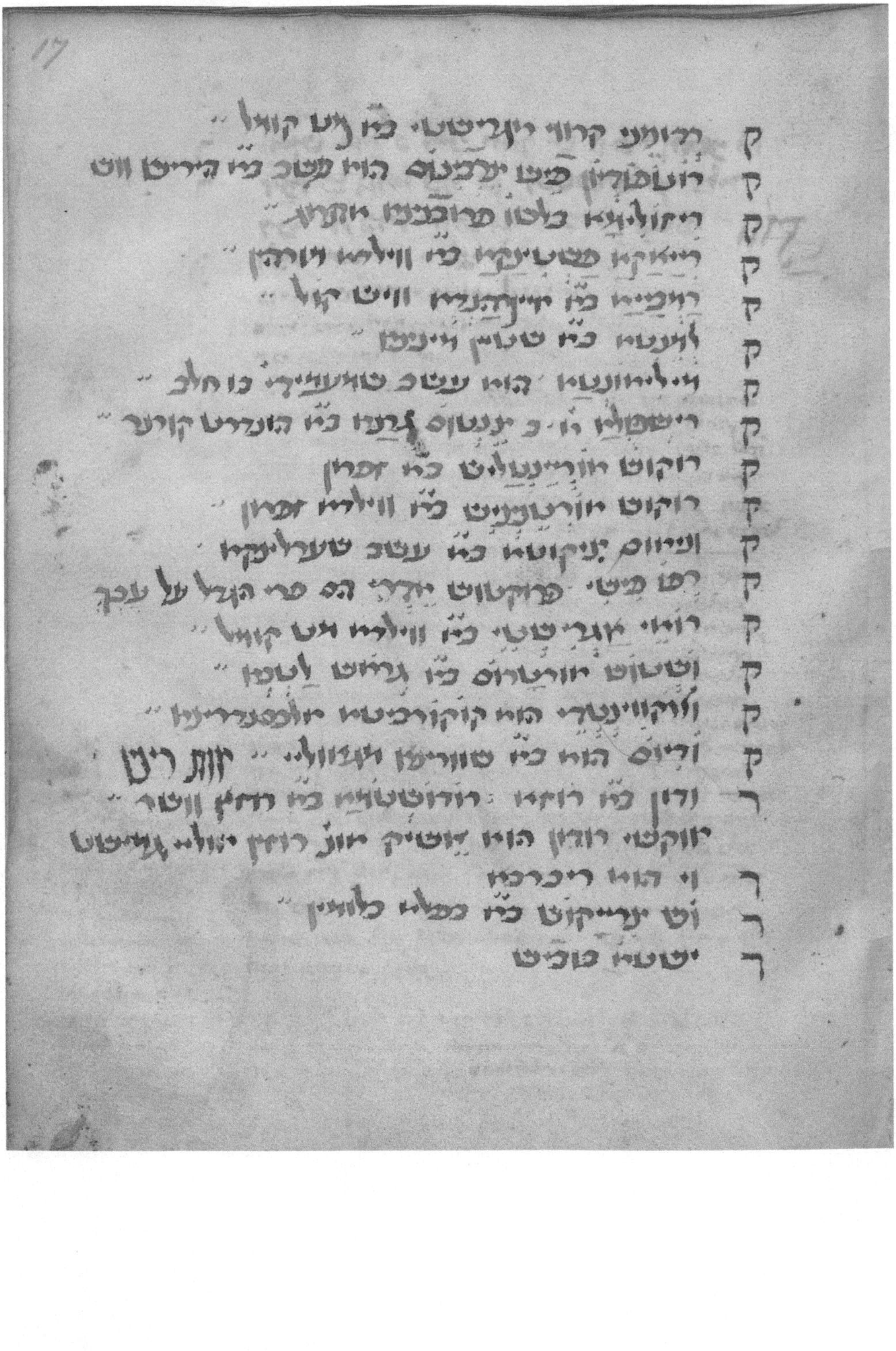

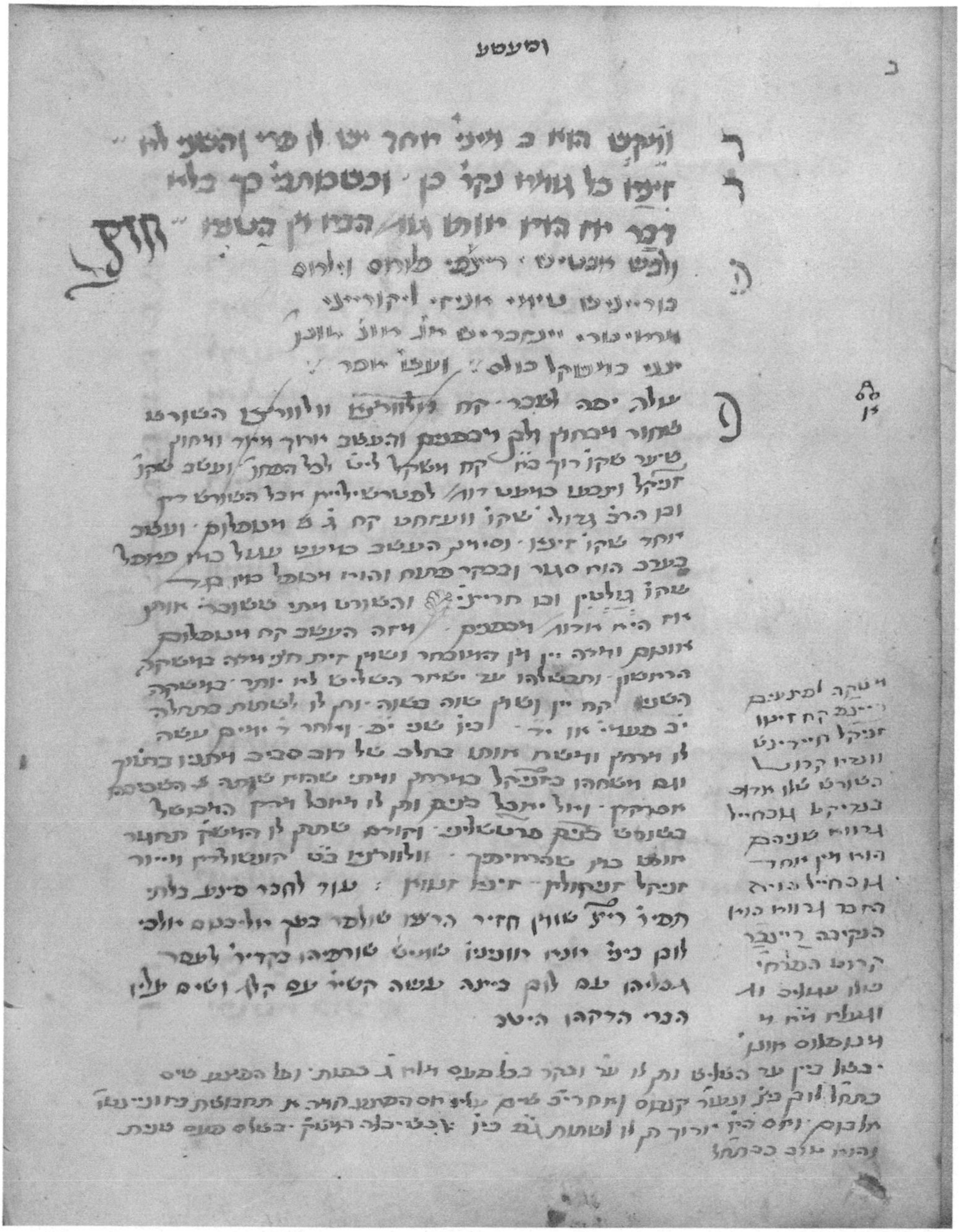

Printed in the United States
By Bookmasters